Biographical Memoirs
Book Three
Physicians, Volume I, 1787–1935

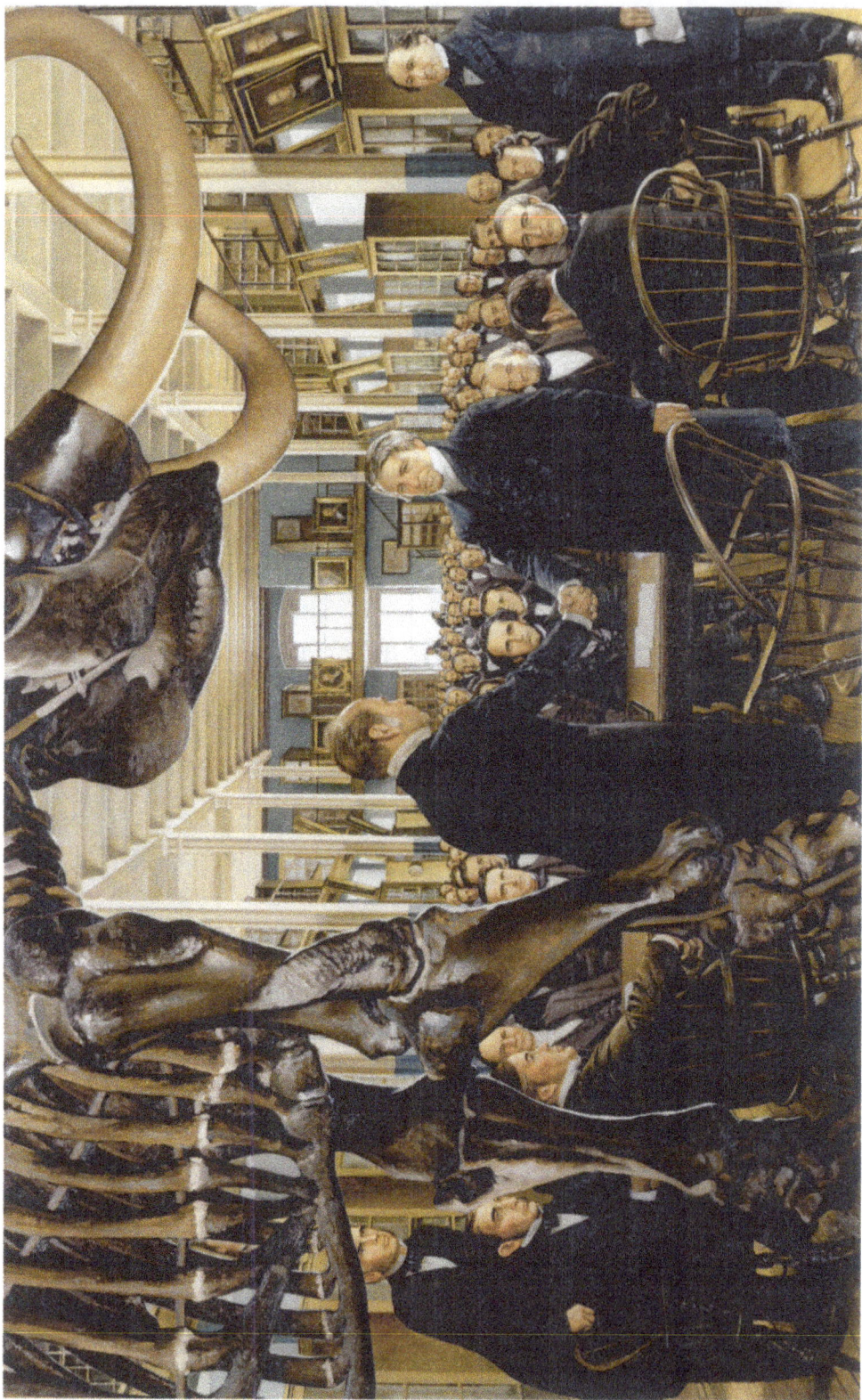

Robert Thom, United States, 1915–1979
"Founding Fathers of the American Medical Association"
Oil on Canvas, 163.83 cm. x 133.35 cm. (64.5 in. x 52.5 in.)
Collection of the University of Michigan Health System,
Gift of Pfizer Inc. UMHS.27

APS Physicians in the Evolution of U.S. Medical Education

Featured in this collection are the memoirs of many of the physicians responsible for the development of modern American medical education. Depicted in this painting is a signal event in this process, the founding meeting of the American Medical Association (AMA).

In the early American colonies there were no medical schools. Anyone could call himself a doctor and practice medicine regardless of lack of education or experience. With the support and encouragement of Benjamin Franklin and John Fathergill the first American medical schools were founded. The first ones were at universities, e.g. the College of Philadelphia (University of Pennsylvania) in 1765, Kings College (Columbia) in 1767 and Harvard in 1782. Later other schools sprang up that were independent of universities or colleges, mostly with disastrous results. The majority of these were proprietary schools lacking adequate faculties or facilities for clinical teaching. Since no accreditation body or process existed, these diploma mills proliferated so that by the 1840s medical education in the U.S. was in chaos.

The first concerted effort at improving and standardizing U.S. medical education was made in 1847 at the founding meeting of the American Medical Association. This first national medical convention was organized by a New York physician, Nathan Smith Davis, but APS physicians from Philadelphia played a prominent role.

The painting by Robert A. Thom on the opposite page depicts this meeting which was held in Philadelphia at the Academy of Natural Sciences. With the ancient bones of a mastodon looking on, APS President Nathaniel Chapman (p. 20) is being congratulated on his election as the AMA's first president. Four of the new Association's eight officers were APS members. APS physicians Isaac Hays, George B. Wood and Alfred Stillé are sitting at the right end of the table.

Proposed at the AMA's founding meeting were elevated standards for medical school admission and graduation and for licensing of physicians. However enactment of these recommendations would take almost another century. Even at university schools, faculty members opposed them, anticipating loss of autonomy and a decline in student enrollment and tuition fees. During subsequent decades as the AMA worked to bring about reform, eleven APS members served as its president. The memoirs of six of them are in this volume (Chapman, Hays, Wood, Gross, Keen and Welch).

Elevation of standards at Penn in 1877 by William Pepper Jr. (p. 105), and in 1893 at Johns Hopkins' new medical school by Welch (p. 144) set the example for improvements but were implemented by few schools. In 1904 the AMA's Council on Medical Education induced the Carnegie Foundation to sponsor a comprehensive survey of U.S. medical schools. The resultant Flexner Report of 1910, by exposing their abuses, caused many of the worst schools to close. Standards first proposed at the founding meeting of the AMA in 1847 were not fully enforced until 1942, when the Liaison Committee of the AMA and the Association of American Medical Colleges was empowered to accredit medical schools.

Biographical Memoirs
of Members of the
American Philosophical Society

Book Three
Physicians, Volume I
Elected 1787–1935

Editors
Clyde F. Barker, Thomas E. Starzl

Biographical Memoirs
of the Members of the
American Philosophical Society

Book Three
Physicians, Volume I
Elected 1787–1935

Biographical Memoirs originally appeared in the
Yearbook of the American Philosophical Society and in the
Proceedings of the American Philosophical Society.

Executive Officer: Keith Thomson
Essay Selection: Clyde F. Barker, Thomas E. Starzl
Editor: Mary McDonald
Associate Editor: Susan Babbitt
Assistant Editors: Dorothy J. Perkins, Herman Baron
Layout and Design: Julie Tipton

Cover Illustration Credits:
Philip Syng Physick, University of Pennsylvania.
Samuel D. Gross, detail from Portrait of Dr. Samuel D. Gross,
  (The Gross Clinic), 1875, by Thomas Eakins.
Harvey Cushing, from The Alan Mason Chesney Medical Archives
  of The Johns Hopkins Medical Institutions.
Casper Wisar, Public domain.
Elisha Kent Kane, United States Postal Service Arctic Explorers
  commemorative stamp, issued May 1986 (no longer in print).

**Sketches are printed in the order in which each Member was elected to
  the American Philosophical Society.

Biographical Memoirs of Members of the
American Philosophical Society
Book Three, Volume I:
Physicians, 1787 to 1935

CONTENTS

Note: Dates indicate the year the physician was inducted as a Member of the APS.

FOREWORD

The American Philosophical Society, the first learned society in North America, has played an important role in American cultural and intellectual life for more than 250 years.

The APS was founded by Benjamin Franklin in 1743 for the purpose of promoting "useful knowledge"—a mission that stands to this day. Early members concentrated on producing research, inventions, and experiments that would "improve the common Stock of Knowledge…to the benefit of Mankind in general."

Since the Society's beginnings, its elected membership has reflected the depth and breadth of scientific and humanistic inquiry, across disciplines and national boundaries. There have been more than 5,000 members since 1743, including men and women who may or may not be household names but whose achievements have been profound.

The American Philosophical Society has had until 1937 a somewhat inconsistent approach to noting the deaths of its Members. What might be read was not always recorded and what was recorded was not always published. Before the institution of the Yearbook only about 200 memoirs were published. Between 1937 and 1991, however, 960 memoirs appeared in the Yearbook and since then, more than 400 have appeared in the Proceedings.

The Committee on Publications has found that many of these obituaries, often written by close colleagues or good friends of the deceased, make for delightful reading. The Committee has decided to invite several Members in a Class to select some of the more readable memoirs in a well populated discipline and bind them together in the hope that they might be of interest to Members and to other scholars in the selected field.

As so many of our Members, especially in the early years, have been physicians, it is not surprising that collecting, editing, and publishing their obituaries (memoirs) eventually will take three volumes. We all are grateful to two eminent physicians, our President Dr. Clyde F. Barker (Class II, 1997) and his colleague Dr. Thomas E. Starzl (Class II, 1999), for taking on this task. Our thanks also to Mary McDonald and Susan Babbitt, editors, and Herman Baron of Diane Publishing, for facilitating the publication.

Keith Thomson
American Philosophical Society Executive Officer
APS Member, Class II (2011)

INTRODUCTION

This is the first of three planned volumes of APS memoirs of Society members who were physicians. It contains the necrologies of 34 members elected between 1787 and 1935. Volumes II and III will contain the memoirs of physician members.

Remarkably, we can recognize the foundation of much of modern scientific medicine in the accounts of these early physicians written by their friends. In addition to their practice, many of these doctors had substantial non-medical interests and activities, and some made significant contributions to the "outside" fields. Their broad interests reflected the young country's fascination during the 19th century with dinosaurs, the languages and customs of the Native Americans, and the study and photography of heavenly bodies such as the moon and the Transit of Venus. There also was romance and adventure: a ship's surgeon and future APS member captured by pirates in the China Sea and then escaping; the icebound winter of a physician/celebrity hero searching the Arctic for the fabled Northwest Passage.

Of some 5,000 Society members elected since its founding in 1743, several hundred have been physicians. With a complete collection of their memoirs, one could chart the entire progress in medicine during that period. That was not our purpose. Instead, we followed the lead of the first two publications in this series (APS classicists and chemists) and selected memoirs that we hoped would make enjoyable reading while providing insight into the personalities, accomplishments, disappointments, and eccentricities of the medical heroes.

Our task was made less daunting by the fact that an APS memoir was never published for many of the doctors. In compliance with the guidelines for this series, we did not borrow memoirs from elsewhere or write new ones even though this meant leaving out important physicians. Although most of the memoirs are faithful reproductions, a few that were excessively long required shortening for inclusion. In three instances, this was done by the APS Library staff rather than by a fellow APS member or a friend.

We decided not to republish memoirs of any of the 53 physicians for whom a complete biographical sketch appeared in Whitfield Bell's and Charles Greifenstein's *Patriot-Improvers*, which reviewed the lives of all 281 APS members from the years 1743 to 1768. These included Benjamin Rush, John Morgan, William Shippen, Thomas Bond, Cadwallader Colden, Samuel Bard, John Redman, and Adam Kuhn.

There are no foreign members in our collection since honorary members during our period of study rarely took part in APS meetings or had memoirs written. Thus, iconic APS members such as John Hunter, Edward Jenner, Claude Bernard, Henry Dale, John Fothergill, Joseph Lister, William Roentgen, Karl Rokitansky, and Rudolf Virchow are notable by their absence.

Other doctors whose memoirs were among the 130 that were available were left out because of space limitations, because the quality of their memoirs was substandard, or because the member's contributions to medicine or to the APS were at the low end of the scale. In essence, the most important criteria for inclusion were the interest and quality of the memoir.

Important physicians on the omitted list, some of whom had no memoir, include John Shaw Billings, S. Weir Mitchell, Oliver Wendall Holmes, D. Hayes Agnew, Austin Flint, Henry Pancoast, Chevalier Jackson, John Collins Warren, Rosewell Park, William Gorgas, Christian Fanger, Jacob Bigalow, Roger Wolcott Sperry, William Sydney Thayer, Franklin Mall, Eli Kennedy Marshall,

Samuel Meltzer, Robley Dunglison, John Charles DaCosta, Alfred Stille, Joseph Carson, John Ashurst, Charles Bingham Penrose, William Horner, David Linn Edsall, Hideyo Noguchi, William B. MacNider, William T. Councilman, John H. Brinton, Henry Boditch, William DeWeese, James Tyson, William Jacobs, Nathaniel Archer Randolph, John Adams Ryder, R.A.F. Penrose, James C. Wilson, Thomas McCray, Alexander Craven Abbot, Edward Martin, Frederick Tilney, Alfred Stengel, George de Schweinitz, Albert H. Smith, Thomas Kirkbride, James E. Rhoads, Thomas G. Morton, Edward Rhoads, John Forsythe Meigs, John L. Leconte, William McIlvaine, and Charles W. Short. Testimony to the prominence and importance of these famous doctors is given by the ready accessibility of their life histories in Wikipedia, the *Encyclopedia Britannica,* or *Biographical Memoirs of the National Academy of Sciences.*

Notwithstanding the omission of so many great contributors to medical science, it is possible from the selected memoirs to piece together the stories behind epochal medical advances of this early era.

Antisepsis: There is no memoir on the originator of antiseptic surgery (honorary APS member Joseph Lister), but W.W. Keen (p. 126) is credited as the first American surgeon to apply it. Denial of importance of antisepsis by Samuel D. Gross (p. 82), America's most influential surgeon, helped delay its use in America for many years. Charles Meigs (p. 35) also opposed antisepsis, and ridiculed Oliver Wendell Holmes (APS 1888, no memoir) for suggesting that if obstetricians washed their hands, many deaths from childbirth fever would be prevented.

Anesthesia: None of the four Americans credited for the origins of ether anesthesia were elected to APS. The foreign member James Y. Simpson (APS 1897) originated chloroform anesthesia, and another Englishman, Humphry Davy (APS 1810), recognized even earlier the soporific action of nitrous oxide.

Vascular Surgery: The techniques of vascular Surgery were perfected in animal experiments by Alexis Carrel (p. 162) and utilized for successful transplantation in animals.

Neurosurgery: W.W. Keen (p. 126) was the first to remove a brain tumor with success, but Harvey Cushing (p. 178) gets the credit for making neurosurgery an important surgical specialty.

Blood Transfusion: Karl Landsteiner (p. 183) defined blood groups, allowing blood transfusions to be safely given.

Anticoagulation: W.H. Howell (p. 155) studied blood coagulation and introduced heparin to prevent clotting.

Medical Education: William Welch (p. 144) at the new school, Johns Hopkins, and William Pepper (p. 105) at the University of Pennsylvania established the guidelines for modern medical school education.

Diverse non-medical fields in which these physicians contributed substantially include:

Paleontology: Casper Wistar (p. 1), Joseph Leidy (p. 68), and Isaac Hays (p. 54).

Astronomy and Photography: John W. Draper (p. 64) and Henry Draper (p. 120).

Anthropology, Archaeology, and Ethnology: Daniel Brinton (p. 97).

Polar Exploration: Elisha Kent Kane (p. 73).

A memoir of the most famous APS doctor (Dr. Benjamin Franklin) does not appear in this collection. Ben Franklin never claimed to be a physician and was called Dr. Franklin only after 1759, when he was awarded an honorary doctorate from Saint Andrews University in Scotland for his work on electricity. But as a natural philosopher and experimentalist he was intensely interested in the medicine of his time and a participant in it. He studied the effectiveness of smallpox vaccinations, causes of the common cold, and lead poisoning. He invented bifocal glasses and evaluated electric shock for treatment of palsies and mental disorders. With his APS colleagues he helped found the first American hospital and medical school. He would have been fascinated to read in this volume the stories of his successors. Hopefully, present-day members of the Society and others will find them interesting.

Clyde F. Barker
President, American Philosophical Society
Former John Rhea Burton Professor
 and Chairman
Donald Guthrie Professor
Department of Surgery
Hospital of the University of Pennsylvania
APS Member, Class II (1997)

Thomas E. Starzl
Professor of Surgery
University of Pittsburgh School
 of Medicine
APS Member, Class II (1999)

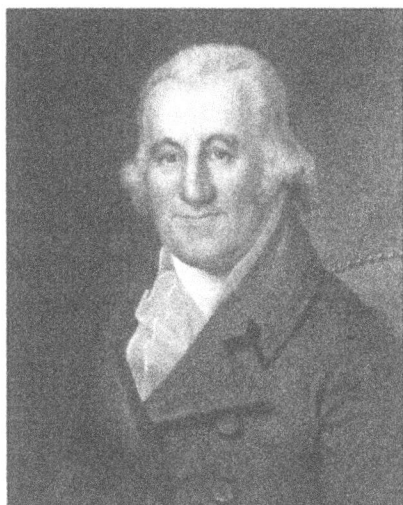

CASPAR WISTAR

1761–1818 (APS 1787)

Memoir by APS Library staff

Caspar Wistar (1761–1818, APS 1787) was a Philadelphia physician and paleontologist. He was a professor at the University of Pennsylvania for three decades, and he served the American Philosophical Society in various offices, including that of president. He was the host of the popular weekly gatherings of local and visiting learned men that became known as the Wistar Parties.

He was born in Philadelphia, the son of Richard Wistar (1727–1781), a glass manufacturer, and Sarah Wyatt Wistar (1733–1771). His seven siblings included his younger sister Catharine, who was married to Benjamin Franklin's grandson William Bache. Wistar is sometimes called Caspar Wistar Jr. to distinguish him from his grandfather, also named Caspar Wistar (1696–1752). The elder Caspar was a merchant and glassmaker who had moved from Wald-Hilspach, Germany, to Philadelphia in 1717.

Born a Quaker, Wistar was educated at the Friends School at Fourth and Walnut Streets in Philadelphia. At age sixteen he volunteered as a nurse at the Battle of Germantown in 1777. It is said that this experience inspired him to become a physician. He commenced his medical studies that year, under the physician John Redman (APS) and later also with John Jones (APS), a New York physician who had fled to Philadelphia. In 1779 Wistar enrolled in the medical department of what was then called the University of the State of Pennsylvania. In 1782, after receipt of his bachelor of medicine, he set out for a three year tour of study in England and Scotland. (Wistar was a practicing Friend throughout his life; however, prior to his departure he had trouble securing a certificate that testified to his diligent adherence to conduct becoming to a Friend, for he had fallen "into scandalous & alarming temptation of being engaged in a duel.") While still a student he was elected one of the presidents of

1

the Royal Medical Society and also president of the Society for the Further Investigation of Natural History. During his stay in England and Scotland he made the acquaintance of several notable figures, including James Boswell, Sir James McIntosh and William Cullen (1710–1790, APS 1768). In 1786 he graduated from the University of Edinburgh with a doctorate of medicine.

Back in Philadelphia, Wistar established a private medical practice that soon grew into one of the largest in the city. He was also elected to the College of Physicians and served as a physician to the Philadelphia Dispensary. In 1788 he became a professor of chemistry at the medical school of the College of Philadelphia. After the merger of the College with the University of the State of Pennsylvania in 1791, Wistar became an adjunct professor of anatomy, midwifery, and surgery. In 1793 he joined the staff of the Pennsylvania Hospital. He nearly lost his life during the yellow fever epidemic of 1793 after being stricken by the disease while assisting his friend Benjamin Rush (1745–1813, APS 1768) in fighting the epidemic. Differences of opinion regarding treatment of this disease, including the drastic use of bleeding and purging, eventually caused a breach in their friendship. Nevertheless, Wistar remained Rush's colleague at the Pennsylvania Hospital until 1810. In 1808 he was appointed to the chair in anatomy that had formerly been occupied by William Shippen. Wistar remained on the Penn faculty until his death in 1818.

Wistar was a popular teacher who enlivened his presentations with drawings and models that made it easier for students to follow his lectures and demonstrations. He developed a number of unique teaching aids, some of which were life-sized anatomical models made of dried and wax-injected human limbs and organs. Others were fashioned of wood, carved by America's first professional sculptor, William Rush. Two years before his death, Wistar appointed Dr. William Edmonds Horner (1793–1853, APS 1819), his long-time assistant in anatomy, as caretaker of these valuable models. Horner later enlarged the collection and opened the first anatomical museum in the United States, the Wistar and Horner Museum. The collection eventually passed to the Wistar Institute of Anatomy and Biology, the first independent medical research facility established in the United States. The Institute, which was founded in 1892 by Wistar's great-nephew, Isaac J. Wistar (1827–1905, APS 1893), was named in honor of Caspar Wistar.

Wistar's reputation drew medical students to Philadelphia from around the world. His anatomy courses became so large that they eventually had to be divided into sections. Wistar wrote the first and very successful treatise on anatomy published in the United States, titled *A System of Anatomy* (2 vols., 1811, 1814). However, he was widely respected not only for his medical knowledge, but also for his general breadth of knowledge, which included the humanities as well as the sciences. In fact, while Wistar made few contributions to medical literature—his only medical article, a description of the sphenoid sinuses, was published the year he died—he contributed several papers on scientific subjects outside of medicine, including paleontology and botany. His reputation as an authority on fossil bones was established as early as 1787, when he and Timothy Matlack (1730–1823, APS 1780) presented a paper on what may have been the first dinosaur bone examined by American scientists. In 1799 he published an article on the bones of the giant "megalonix" that Thomas Jefferson had deposited with the American Philosophical Society two years earlier. The essay, which appeared in the Society's *Transactions*, is regarded as the first technical study of professional quality to be published by an American or in America in the field of vertebrate paleontology. One historian has called the achievement "almost incredible in view of the paleontological naïveté of his associates and of the lack of comparative materials." Wistar also collaborated in Jefferson's efforts to obtain the bones of the mastodon and associated animals, and he studied specimens returned from the Lewis and Clark Expedition. Some of his observations on the latter were published posthumously in the *Transactions*.

Wistar was as popular with his professional colleagues as he was with Philadelphia's literati. He was particularly known for his hospitality, and his home was the weekly meeting place of students and scientists, including locals and distinguished foreign visitors. The physician Charles Caldwell (1772–1853, APS 1796) recalled later that "the company met, without ceremony, on a stated evening, where in the midst of a succession of suitable refreshments, the time passed away, oftentimes until a late hour, in agreeable, varied, and instructive discourse." The "company" included, for example, Alexander von Humboldt (1769–1859, APS 1804), who was a guest of honor when he visited Philadelphia in 1800, as well as the French botanist François Andre Michaux (1749–1802). A frequent attendant after his arrival in the United States in 1812 was the Abbé Corrêa da Serra (1750–1823, APS 1812), the Portuguese diplomat and naturalist. Wistar, who shared with the Abbé a serious interest in botany, became his close friend and accompanied him on several expeditions. The Wistar Parties were so popular that several leading members of the American Philosophical Society, including Stephen DuPonceau (1760–1844, APS 1791), continued to host them regularly after Wistar's death.

Wistar was active in numerous scientific and learned organizations. He was elected to the American Philosophical Society in 1787. He served as its curator in 1793 and vice-president in 1795, before succeeding Thomas Jefferson as president in 1815, a position he held until his death. Wistar was especially supportive of the Historical and Literary Committee that was established in 1815 to serve as the collection, research, and publishing arm of the Society. He was elected a Fellow of the College of Physicians in 1788, and he served as a trustee of the College of Philadelphia from 1789 to 1791. In 1815 he was elected an honorary member of the Literary and Philosophical Society of New York. The botanist Thomas Nuttall (1786–1859, APS 1817) honored Wistar by naming the plant genus *Wisteria* after him.

Wistar's support of many progressive causes is reflected in his affiliation with a number of reform organizations. He was a founder of the Society for Circulating the Benefit of Vaccination, and he belonged to the Pennsylvania Prison Society, the Humane Society, and the Society for the Abolition of Slavery, of which he became president in 1813. In 1791 Wistar bought and then freed a slave "to extricate him from that degraded Situation."

Caspar Wistar died in 1818 after a period of declining health. He was married twice, first in 1788 to Isabella Marshall, who died childless two years later. In 1798 he married Elizabeth Mifflin, with whom he had three children: Dr. Richard Mifflin Wistar, Dr. Mifflin Wistar, and Elizabeth Wistar. There were no grandchildren.

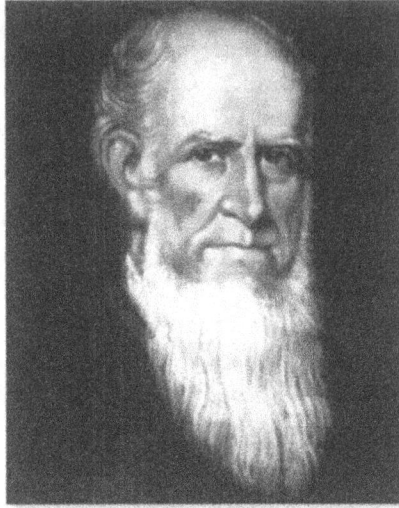

CHARLES CALDWELL

1772–1853 (APS 1796)

Memoir by Benjamin H. Coates

Charles Caldwell was born about 1772, in Caswell, then a part of Orange county, North Carolina. There exists abundant and uncontradicted evidence that he very soon gave proof of a superior under-standing. He studied perseveringly, both at school and at home; and made very rapid progress. From eleven to fourteen he studied Latin and some Greek; retaining the high estimation which had been conceded to him by his fellow scholars. At fourteen, he states that he was thought not likely to im-prove further by a continuance at any school then extant in North Carolina; and, before the end of his fifteenth year, he was called upon to discharge the office of conducting academies for the instruction of others. In this there exists copious evidence that he met with brilliant success. In the meanwhile, he made use of the assistance of a neighboring clergyman, to prosecute a short mathematical and physical course.

His preference, in the choice of a permanent profession, was for law or for the army; and a com-mission was offered him. His father was now deceased; but had always entertained a strong dislike to his son's adoption of either of these two modes of life; and Mr. Caldwell, in consequence of this, determined to apply himself to medicine. In the spring of 1791, he entered the office of Dr. Harris, of Salisbury, North Carolina; and, in the autumn of 1792, repaired to Philadelphia. Here he devoted himself, with great industry, to study, and to attendance on lectures and on the Pennsylvania Hospital. During the great epidemic of yellow fever, in 1793, he had and used great opportunities for obser-vation in that terrible disease; and formed or founded some of the convictions for which he became afterwards conspicuous. He passed examinations in medicine in 1794, his name is inserted in the list of graduates in 1795, but did not take out his diploma till 1796; a delay which arose from pecuniary losses. His thesis is theoretical; and develops some of the opinions of Dr. Rush. His career, as an author, opened with his translations of Blumenbach's *Physiology*, in 1794; and continued for sixty years!

In the autumn of 1794, finding his health materially injured by his application, Dr. Caldwell became a surgeon in the army raised to suppress the Whiskey Insurrection. This, as is well known, was happily, and in consonance with the anxious wishes of President Washington, terminated without bloodshed. The march through the forest completely restored our young fellow member to his health; and, in 1796, he commenced practice in Philadelphia.

In 1797, the yellow fever of that year first broke out in the vicinity of Dr. Caldwell's residence. Many physicians, it is notorious, fled from their posts before the formidable pestilence; but Dr. Caldwell remained. A vehement controversy arose on the questions whether the disease were contagious, and whether it were of foreign or domestic origin. The effects of these two controversies, after a lapse of near sixty years, have by no means ceased to be felt among our citizens. Numerous pens were occupied with assaults, often violent, upon that eminent teacher, Dr. Rush; and these were by no means restrained from his practice as a therapeutist.

Dr. Caldwell, early in 1778, adopted and earnestly defended a belief in the domestic origin of the fever; and much of his very animated discussions is to be found in the newspapers. The therapeutics of Dr. Rush met with his warm and earnest support; as he alleges that he found them the most successful in practice.

It is well known that Dr. Rush, though an early believer in the domestic origin of the disease, was at first persuaded that it was contagious. In this he was opposed by Dr. Physick; who, however, took part in no public controversies, but confined the expression of his opinions to friends and intimates, and sometimes replied to inquirers in monosyllables, attending closely, at the same time, to his labours as a practitioner. Dr. Rush, as is familiar to tradition and to reading, subsequently changed his mind in relation to the existence of such a contagion; but Dr. Caldwell preceded him by a considerable interval; and, at one time, the last named physician was singly associated, among all his intimates, with Dr. Physick.

At length, Dr. Caldwell was himself stricken down with the pestilence; and was recovered, after an illness of three weeks, by the skill and care of Drs. Physick and Rush, and by the indefatigable attentions of his friend and fellow student, Dr. Samuel Cooper, of Delaware. In the course of the two subsequent epidemics, of 1801 and 1803, he describes himself as having been, what has been so often denied to exist, an example of repeated attacks in the same individual. Through the fatal and terrific visitation of 1798, and through those of 1799 and 1805, he passed uninjured.

In 1798, the first Academy of Medicine was founded. The long and ardent discussions in which the members of this body engaged, are well recollected by readers and survivors. The Academy, though short-lived, endured sufficiently long to publish a large amount of matter against the contagious character of yellow fever.

Between 1805 and 1807, Dr. Caldwell delivered the first course of clinical lectures in the medical department of the Philadelphia Almshouse, now the Blockley Hospital. Besides large contributions to the medical journals, he was the author of various eulogiums and other addresses. In the winter of 1810-11, he prepared and read a series of lectures on medical jurisprudence, simultaneously with that by Dr. Stringham, in New York; these forming the two first courses ever delivered in this country. Dr. Caldwell's course was several times repeated.

Between 1800 and 1811 he prepared a very large amount of manuscript, chiefly lectures and controversial matter; the total amount of writing which he has left behind him being estimated by a female connection at thirty thousand pages. During this period, too, his literary correspondence became large.

In 1815, the Physical Faculty of the University of Pennsylvania was created; and Dr. Caldwell was made professor of geology and the philosophy of natural history. He delivered three courses. Soon after this period, Dr. Caldwell was invited to take part in the establishment of three new medical schools, in New York, Philadelphia, and Baltimore. These he declined; but, in 1819, accepted an invitation to unite in the formation of Transylvania University, at Lexington, Kentucky; and to occupy the professorship of the Institutes of Medicine. To these tasks he devoted himself with all ardour; and to the extent of making much personal sacrifice. "It is not too much to affirm, says Dr. L. P. Yandell, "that he was the father of the Western School of Medicine." Dr. Caldwell's exertions mainly contributed to obtain, from the Legislature of Kentucky, the requisite funds to procure a library and apparatus; and he himself visited Europe to watch the proper expenditure. The character of the institution became high, the connection influential, and the class large.

During the creation of a new school, at Louisville, in the same State, and the transfer of legislative patronage to it, Dr. Caldwell relates, in his MS., that he resisted the change till he became convinced that it was inevitable, and then added his activity to the new institution. This was from love of science and mankind, and from the duty of patriotism, as a good citizen submits to an already accomplished revolution. Even here, too, he is pronounced by competent authority, to have become entitled, by effective labour and personal influence, to be considered also a founder.

His services were eminently great and active during the first few years; and he was far from intermitting his literary toils. He continued to support those heavy burdens till 1849; when, at 77 years of age, he resigned his professorship. During this period, the influence of the new school slowly and steadily increased; and the numbers of the class reached four hundred. During the last years of his life, our fellow-member continued in the enjoyment of uninterrupted health, an erect attitude, and the perfect use of his faculties. The termination of his earthly existence occurred, in an almost entire freedom from suffering and disease, on the 9th of July, 1853.

Dr. Caldwell was twice married. In 1799, he was united to Eliza, daughter of Thomas Leaming, Esq., of Philadelphia. By this lady, he has left one son, Dr. Thomas Leaming Caldwell, of Louisville, Kentucky. His second matrimonial connection was with Mrs. Barton, the youngest daughter of the late honourable William Warner, of the State of Delaware, and related to several eminent citizens of that commonwealth. This union was without offspring.

He received several compliments from the European learned, but was careless of his diplomas; and a list cannot be made out. His election to the American Philosophical Society took place October 21, 1796.

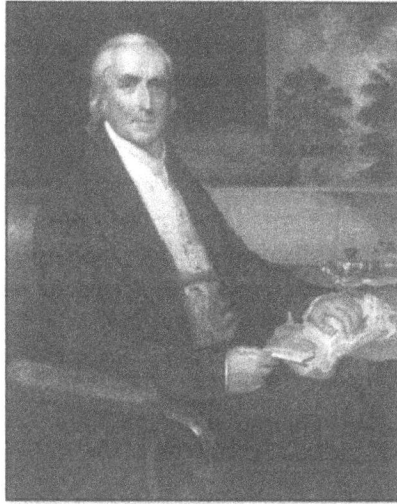

PHILIP SYNG PHYSICK

1768–1837 (APS 1802)

Memoir by William E. Horner

The unique 32-page obituary of Dr. Philip Syng Physick cannot be fully understood without knowing more about its author, William Edmonds Horner (1793–1853). Although Dr. Horner was a long-standing member of the Society and had prepared another obituary (for a W.S. Jacobs), his own death notice could not be found. Eventually, a collection of Horner memorabilia donated in 1974 by his great-grandson (Dr. Albert R. Shands) was discovered in the University of Pennsylvania Archives and Records Center. These files together with statements contained in the final two paragraphs of his Physick obituary make it possible to better understand what Dr. Horner had written about Dr. Physick's life and death.

Penultimate Obituary Paragraph...And it is known to yourselves that the present memoir *[Physick's obituary]* is the result of respectful sentiments on the part of the American Philosophical Society: of sentiments arising rather from the intercourse of the sick chamber, and the confidence of private life, than from any signal contribution on the part of the subject of it, to the objects of the Society. We can, however, scarcely doubt that, with a larger share of health, and fewer pressing engagements, we should have seen him, like our lamented President, Wistar, exciting, by his frequent presence, the zeal of the Society, and giving a direction to its enterprise. The example and the lessons of his great master, Hunter, had certainly prepared him well for such an exertion of his talents in physiology and comparative anatomy.

Material in Bold Italic has been added by co-editor Thomas E. Starzl

In other words, Dr. Physick apparently played no role in the affairs of the American Philosophical Society after his election to membership in 1802 at the age of 34. There is no hint whether this was simply due to his lack of time or had some more personal explanation.

Final Obituary Paragraph…In carrying this notice probably beyond the intention of the original resolution, the usage of the Society, and also beyond those bounds to which I could with propriety trust myself, as defining my own competency and your feeling of patience, I have this apology to offer:—The relation subsisting between myself and the individual, whose traits and virtues I have so imperfectly commemorated, was one of ardent affection on my part—of profound veneration—of benefits received, and few, perhaps none returned;—of a kindness which took me by the hand, at a time when I was youthful and unpatronized; and by its activity and uniform tenour, infused encouragement, strengthened the imbecility of early professional life, and finally led to whatever may be most valuable in my condition.

What occurred in Dr. Horner's life that so indebted him to Dr. Physick? Horner's private education and apprenticeship resembled that of other APS members who were physicians. After service in a military hospital during the War of 1812, he began his career at the University of Pennsylvania in 1816 as a dissector under Caspar Wistar. Six years later, he was appointed dean of the medical school, a post that he held for 30 years (1822–1852), while doubling up between 1831 and 1851 as Dr. Physick's successor in the chair of anatomy. His Treatise on Pathological Anatomy *was the first American textbook on this subject. As one of the primary architects of the evolving medical school, he advanced the interests of his faculty with particular emphasis on the largely unpublished accomplishments of his older-by-25-years idol, Professor Physick. More than any other person, he shaped Dr. Physick's iconography and ultimate apotheosis. His determination to present a multidimensional description of Dr. Physick is explicitly stated in the Preamble of the obituary.*

NECROLOGICAL NOTICE
Of
DR. PHILIP SYNG PHYSICK

The decision of the Society having committed to me the difficult task of portraying the attributes and character of one of its most illustrious and gifted members, I now discharge the duty with a consciousness of much inability to do it justice. Great men and great mountains should be seen from a distance, in order to appreciate their exact magnitude and their relation to surrounding objects; proximity of the eye enables us to view more distinctly the various productions and undulations of surface, but disqualifies to an equal degree from seizing upon those bold comparative features, which give the liveliest interest to narrative of every kind.

The duty of the biographer is moreover intrinsically difficult: on the one hand he has to rescue from oblivion the characteristic thoughts, habits, and actions of the individual he commemorates, and to present such of his traits as may possibly become the incentive and guide to others: on the other hand, to render the picture complete, and thereby to avoid a strain of mere compliment, he has to furnish those incidents and points which reduce the hero and the sage to the mere man; and in doing so runs the risk of a background too somber or too uniform, for the due reflection of features which he desires to make prominent. Where in addition personal attachment exists, our predisposition to favour great men makes us eulogize their virtues and strong points, and suppress the narrative of weaknesses and peculiarities: yet much of the interest which attaches to them upon moral and philosophical grounds, depends upon a knowledge of both sides of the question. Among the most striking incidents in the history of Caesar is his dissoluteness and prodigality in early life, and his infatuation for Cleopatra when he became the head of the Roman Empire: but none among us would be pleased with the historian who, from tenderness to his memory, should suppress the narrative of these events. On the same ground how much would we lose by not knowing that Alexander the Great, on the occasion of a feast, had in a paroxysm of intemperate rage plunged a dagger into the bosom of his most esteemed and veteran general Clitus, and had finally died suddenly in Babylon in a drunken revel.

Neither has the inspired volume spared its great men: it records that to Moses, the chosen servant of God, and the leader of his people, it was said, "Go up into that mountain and die there, thou shalt see from thence the land that I will give to the children of Israel, but thou shalt not enter it; because you transgressed against me at the waters of contradiction, and did not sanctify me among the children of Israel." Deut. xxxi. 50. The same volume has not failed to narrate distinctly the licentiousness of David, nor the tergiversation of Solomon; and this candor gives it additional recommendation to the scholar. Why then, it may be asked, with these venerable examples of antiquity before it, should modern biography be a eulogy, instead of an exposition of character? In the case of the obscure and unimportant individual, whether in high life or in low life, the ephemeral tribute of praise may, in the form of an obituary notice, be all incense; it does no harm, for we understand it as the effusion of some attached friend, whose grief finds its solace in this expression of it. Such comment is not documentary, and the unmarked life of the individual is soon buried in oblivion.

This however is not the case in one of Nature's master-pieces. In the man whose genius has impressed the nation or the period when he lived, perfect candor in all the disquisitions concerning him, is the best tribute to his memory. Men whose minds have a strong tendency in one direction, may in all the scrutiny's instituted be found to harmonize their actions according to that cardinal point, but it would be unphilosophical to expect equal force and equal harmony in an opposite direction.

With this preamble I may now proceed to state, that Dr. Philip S. Physick, whose memory we are about to recall, was distinguished by a long and triumphant course in Surgery and Medicine by a deep and universal conviction on the medical and public mind of this country in favor of his skill; and by traits of character so prominent and so peculiar, that the chances are very improbable of their being repeated in any other individual. Even if nature should renew her production, the difference of circumstances in which it will be placed, from the immense changes constantly and rapidly occurring in our social state, will prevent the same mode and degree of development.

Born on the 7th of July, 1768, in Third, near Arch Street, Philadelphia; his father, Mr. Edmund Physick, was a native of England; and his mother, Miss Syng, the daughter of a celebrated silversmith of this city, who was one of the early friends and companions of Franklin, and whose name appears on the register of the American Philosophical Society as one of its founders. His maternal grandfather appears to have possessed a large share of practical sense and industry; to have lived much respected; and to have raised a numerous family, among whom he divided a good estate on his death. His character made a strong impression on Dr. Physick's mind: I have frequently heard it quoted by him, with veneration, as a good example of what a proper course in life will accomplish.

At the breaking out of the Revolutionary War, Mr. Physick, the father, resided with his family in the Valley of Chester County, Pennsylvania. Governor John Penn, being deposed by the colony then in arms, was ordered from his estate of Lansdowne, situated a few miles above Philadelphia on the west side of the Schuylkill, and directed into the interior of New Jersey. Mr. Physick, at the request of Governor Penn, took charge of the Lansdowne estate, and resided upon it at a place called the Hat. This arrangement produced a considerable intimacy between the two families. The estate being on the belligerent line, Mr. Physick received a protection from General Howe, then in Philadelphia, and another from General Washington, then at Valley Forge. It was in the winter of this period that Mr. Physick, on visiting Valley Forge, observed that the cannons of the American army were frozen immovably in the mud; so that if General Howe had made an attack, they could not have been worked.

The subject of our memoir received his academic education from Robert Proud, in "Friends' Academy," and during the time lived in the family of Mr. John Tod, the father-in-law of the present Mrs. Madison. He then entered the classical department of the University of Pennsylvania and obtained his knowledge of the languages from Mr. James Davidson, one of the best scholars of his day. No small fondness for these, his earlier studies, remained with him to the end of his life.

Having passed honorably through his college studies, he received the degree of Bachelor of Arts. His father now considered him ready to engage in the study of medicine, and made a movement to that effect. His own predilections, however, were for a different employment: with an original natural fondness for mechanical arts, which he had at an early period exhibited by making himself a pair of shoes; this partiality was strengthened by the example of his maternal grandfather, who had led an independent and happy life as a silversmith. His father was found inflexible, and placed him under the charge of the late Dr. Adam Kuhn, one of the most learned and successful physicians of that period. I may here observe, in passing, that notwithstanding Dr. Physick's subsequently unequalled reputation in surgery, and the immense fortune that he acquired principally by professional employment, he never lost this early inclination for mechanical pursuits. Even within a short time of his death, in reflecting upon the events of his life, such as his anxieties for the health of others, his professional excitements, and the decrepitude and ravages made on his own constitution by disease, he regretted that he had not been indulged in his love for the business of a silversmith; his impression was, that in securing to himself health and tranquil employment, his life would have been much happier, and a very sufficient measure of success would have attended his efforts.

His first introduction to anatomy excited strongly his aversion and disgust to the profession of medicine—it was the boiling of a skeleton in the Medical College in Fifth street, now the Health Office. He returned home, and implored again his father to relax his resolution: it was all in vain. Finding his father thus inexorable, he took up his medical studies in earnest. The book of the highest reputation at that period, and which was handed to him with the strongest commendations from Dr. Kuhn, was Cullen's first Lines of the Practice of Physic. In his sincerity of character, he thought within himself: This book being so much esteemed, and containing so many profound and well ascertained points of knowledge, I cannot do better than learn the whole of it accurately. He therefore went to work and committed it to memory, presenting thereby a solitary example probably in the history of medicine of this task accomplished; and which appears the more wonderful to us at the present day, from the comparative disuse into which these volumes have fallen.

When twenty years of age, in 1788, his father took him to London, and succeeded in placing him under the direction of Mr. John Hunter, the great surgeon of the day; and now looked upon as the first medical man that the British empire has produced, his posthumous reputation having gone vastly beyond, any that he ever had when alive. Mr. Hunter was no student of the writings of others, but a profound interrogator of nature; he had little or no respect for any other revelations of science, than those made with the dissecting-knife, and under his own observation. The affair being settled that young Mr. Physick was to study under him, the elder Mr. Physick said, "Well, sir, I presume some books will be required for my son, I will thank you to mention them that I may get them." "Here, sir," says Mr. Hunter, "follow me; I will show you the books your son has to study." Mr. Hunter led the way from his study to his dissecting-room, and entering it pointed to several dead bodies. "These are the books," says he, "which your son will learn under my direction; the others are fit for very little." The impression made on the mind of Dr. Physick was durable; he never forgot the remark, especially after committing to memory Cullen's First Lines, as he had done but a short time before in Philadelphia.

Being thus placed in a dissecting-room, he distinguished himself in a short time by his assiduity, and by the neatness and success of his dissections; he became a favorite with Mr. Home, the assistant in the rooms, and also with Mr. Hunter. The confidence and partiality of the latter were exhibited in the year 1790, while he was still a student under him, by Mr. Hunter using great exertions, and successfully, to get him elected house surgeon to St. George's Hospital. Considerable influence was necessary to obtain this post from the number of competitors for it; and also from the disrelish of the British mind for any American, at so short a period after the Revolutionary War. Having been installed, he was looked upon with jealousy and suspicion. The first call for a trial of his skill being a dislocated shoulder, the other residents of the house assembled around him with distrust and sneers at the American stripling. The adjustments being made, the shoulder was in a moment reduced, which convinced the bystanders, that they had mistaken the object of their feelings.

In the year 1791 he received his diploma from the Royal College of Surgeons in London. After which he visited Edinburgh; and having spent a winter there, took out the degree of Doctor of Medicine in the University, in 1792. In the latter part of the same year he returned home, highly instructed in his profession: after having declined offers by his preceptor, Mr. Hunter, of a promising and advantageous kind, for him to settle in London, This course was probably influenced to some degree by his health, which the climate and atmosphere of that metropolis did not suit. His father secured for him an office in Arch Street, near Third, where he began the practice of medicine, as I have often heard him say, with only two shillings and six-pence in his pocket.

Dr. Physick's inability to attract patients during the first year of his practice was exemplified by anecdotes. His anxieties were allayed when:

The year 1793 brought him distinctly and prominently before the public notice. The premonitory indications of a fatal epidemic being on the approach were but too faithfully verified, when, on the 19th of August, the celebrated Rush announced to his fellow-citizens that a malignant and mortal fever, had broken out among them. This startling intelligence, whereby the repose of the public mind was disturbed, was received at first with the agitation and excitement created by some unexpected convulsion of nature: by some it was discredited, and strong indignation expressed against its author. The celerity, however, with which the disease invaded the several walks of life left no room for disputation, and all that remained to be done, was to make the best possible arrangements for its visitation. Among the measures of the day recommended by the College of Physicians on the 26th of August, and carried into immediate effect, was the providing of a large and airy hospital in the neighborhood of the city, for the reception of such poor persons as could not be accommodated with the above advantages in private houses.

The erection of the Bush Hill Hospital was the result of this recommendation, and Dr. Physick, having offered his services, was chosen physician of the same. He left his lodgings in town, entered immediately upon his new duties, and continued in the exercise of them till the disease had passed away. While on this duty, a disposition to insubordination and riot having been exhibited by the inmates of the hospital, he was appointed alderman by Governor Mifflin, so as to meet any emergency with the promptest attention and vigor. An explanation of this civil magistracy may be given, by stating that such was the panic created by the yellow-fever, that no ordinary civil officer could be found hardy enough, to enter the hospital, to enforce order. I have repeatedly heard the doctor say, that when he was sworn in by the mayor (Matthew Clarkson), the latter held off from the precincts of the hospital, and from Dr. Physick, at the greatest distance compatible with hearing, and was happy to be off as soon as possible, when the ceremony was over. He resigned this office at the end of the season, and it returned again to the gentleman who had previously abdicated it, for the express purpose.

In the year 1794 he was appointed a prescribing physician in the Philadelphia Dispensary, and a surgeon to the Pennsylvania Hospital: the public confidence was also exhibited by his practice increasing with no ordinary rapidity.

A recurrence of the yellow-fever as an epidemic, in 1798, led again to a performance of similar duties in the Bush Hill Hospital. The zeal and fidelity, with which he went through these, were recognized in the presentation of some elegant pieces of silver plate. Their cost was upwards of one thousand dollars, and they bear the following inscription: "From the Board of Managers of the Marine and City Hospitals to *Philip Syng Physick, M.D.* This Mark of their respectful Approbation of his Voluntary and Inestimable Services, as Resident Physician at the City Hospital, in the Calamity of 1798."

The yellow fever caused 10,000 deaths, a figure cited by Sir William Osler in his 1921 book, The Evolution of Modern Medicine (pp. 225–232), and attributed by Osler to a monograph published 123 years earlier (Matthew Carey Philadelphia, 1793). The mortality in the recurrent epidemic in 1798 was almost as high. With these horrors behind him and formation of his family ahead, Philip Syng Physick began a 3-decade career that came to a climax with his successful treatment in 1831 of John Marshall, chief justice of the United State Supreme Court.

Dr. Physick's numerous appointments and distinctions included: attending surgeon at the hospital of the Philadelphia Alms House (1801), membership in the American Philosophical Society (1802), founding chair of the new Department of Surgery (1805) and then the chairmanship of the Department of Anatomy that mandated resignation of his surgical chair (1819). Five years after his retirement in 1831 and one year before his death, he was elected in 1836 to the Royal Medical and Chirurgical Society of London.

He never lacked patients after his heroic role in the yellow fever epidemics made him a household name in Philadelphia.

"He was remarkable for the smallness of his charges, and for an indifference to fees; for he frequently gave up large ones when there was no adequate reason for it."…"With this indifference to fees, he was however exceedingly exact when money was received, in the appropriations of it to some productive end: his professional labours sometimes produced twenty thousand dollars a year, and his method in this respect finally yielded a sum of more than half a million of dollars."

Dr. Horner provided lengthy examples of Dr. Physick's intolerance to a patient's opposition or disingenuousness, and of his demand for compliance. In return, he "…scrupulously abided by, and assisted cheerfully in all that was done. When the cure was finished, the esteem which this candour produced made him feel almost as much obliged to the patient as the patient could be to him, and he often spoke of it afterwards with pleasure."

On Sept. 18th, 1800, he was married to Miss Emlen, the daughter of a gentleman of learning, distinction, and wealth, and who belonged to the very respectable Society of Friends. She died in 1820, leaving four children, now alive—two sons and two daughters.

His personal habits were fixed by an unyielding set and durability. He had passed his life in a certain diurnal movement and rotation, any suspension or deviation of which put him to inconvenience. He must have the bed that he was accustomed to; the same food, dressed in the same way. His delicate health made him seek solitude as a refreshment; he was therefore no diner out; had no habits of conviviality; received no company in a familiar way, except now and then the call of a friend. Though not much of a talker himself, he was susceptible of amusement from lively conversation where he was on familiar terms; otherwise he was very reserved, and sometimes impatient of it. He was particularly irritated at prolixity in a patient, and most frequently would not bear it at all; his common defence against it being a few observations of a catechetical kind, and then a declaration that he had learned enough.

He was no traveller, and had no propensity to be such. The wonderful evolution of the social interests of this country, and the vast augmentation of its inhabitants, all took place while he himself was a chief actor; and yet he never seemed to desire to witness with his own eyes, the prodigies which were going on far and near. He went from Philadelphia to London by the straightest route; he went from London to Edinburgh by the straightest route; he returned from Edinburgh to Philadelphia by the straightest route; and he lived and died in Philadelphia, circumscribing his movements to the smallest compass, and only leaving the city on urgent professional calls, excepting that within the last ten or twelve years he spent short periods of time in the summer at a country seat in Maryland, near Port Deposite, for the improvement of his health.

His habits were frugal and economical; he disliked wanton expenditure, and latterly made an exact estimate of the utility of a thing before he bought it.

From 1800 onward, Dr. Physick's interests were largely focused on the University of Pennsylvania School of Medicine, and specifically on his new Department of Surgery (1805-1819) and the more prestigious Department of Anatomy which was the dominant basic science discipline of the time. Elsewhere in the obituary, Dr. Horner noted that "in 1816 Dr. Physick had resigned the place of surgeon in the Pennsylvania Hospital, being succeeded by Dr. Dorsey; and some years previously he had yielded his appointments in the Philadelphia Dispensary, and in the Alms House Infirmary." In 1816, he resigned his surgical Chair in order to replace Caspar Wistar as chairman of the Department Anatomy.

Doctor Physick's traits as a teacher corresponded with other points in his character. His course of surgery, upon which his reputation was founded in an especial manner, was eminently practical and instructive. He did not pretend to range over the whole field of this science, but limited himself to topics of daily occurrence, or at least such as might be expected in the practice of any medical man. Relying upon his own experience and habits of observation, he had but little to do with the opinions of others; he quoted them rarely, and never in such a way as to leave the point unsettled by an array of opposite authorities. His opinions were for the most part founded upon deep reflection, and were decided in one way or another; he never leaned to one side and inclined to other, so as to neutralize his weight; he either admitted entire want of information, or considered himself in possession of the requisite degree of it. This tone of sentiment pervading his lectures they were most eminently didactic, and were listened to with a thorough conviction of his correctness; indeed such was his authority, that it was held almost as indisputable as a revelation—to oppose it was to brand one-self with folly.

13

He was but little of a reader, and therefore had but a very limited acquaintance with medical literature; he decidedly preferred studying everything for himself in the laboratory of nature, beginning his analysis of the human machine in a dissecting-room, and solving the problem of its disorders and their cure in a hospital. The proposition in every disease he considered as limiting itself, to the positive experience, of what had done good and what had done harm. His consultations always assumed this character.

As his opinions were for the most part formed with deliberation, so they were retained with firmness; and they, like his habits, were durable to an extreme. This we may account for, inasmuch as they were never taken up on capricious grounds, but always upon the most scrupulous examination of proof. He required, too, personal proof, such as would satisfy his understanding, through his eyes, his ears, and his touch. Naturally exact, systematic, and persevering, these traits were fully developed by his education and training; hence his character became finally as unchangeable as the stamp on coin, it had neither voluntary power nor susceptibility of alteration: nothing but a fusion like that of metal could have modified it.

Dr. Physick's sufferings of body and mind were referred to by Dr. Horner throughout the obituary. Almost all were related to sequellae of infectious disease encounters: chronic sinusitis (recurrent catarrh), chronic pyelonephritis with stone formation, renal failure, peptic ulcer, and probably the valve disease of rheumatic fever.

During his whole life the subject of this notice had occasionally violent illness. In very early infancy, before he could recollect, he suffered from inoculated small-pox so severely that his life was despaired of; the eruption having passed so far down his throat, as to come near strangling him. The marks of this attack were left on his face in pits, which were somewhat visible to the day of his death.

When in St. George's Hospital he had a severe illness, and was attended there by a female nurse with a degree of fidelity, which made a lasting impression on him. Her goodness and disinterestedness were rendered still more striking, by her declining afterwards to receive compensation, as she considered the duty a part of her obligation to the house.

He had an attack of Yellow-fever in 1793, and another in 1797. The latter went near to destroy him. He told me that, as he lay ill, he could hear through his windows, which were open, a stout blacksmith, who lived near, inquire daily of his black waiter, "Is your master dead yet?" To which the monotonous response of "No !" was as often given. When the doctor recovered sufficiently to leave the house, he inquired after the blacksmith who had so frequently saluted his ears with this disagreeable question. He found that the blacksmith himself, had in the meantime been one of the victims of the epidemic.

In the winter of 1813–14, when the typhus fever prevailed here, he had a severe and protracted attack of it, from which he narrowly escaped. Drs. Kuhn and Wistar attended him. He came out of this sickness much reduced in flesh, and I think never recovered his volume afterwards.

In early life he was subject to bleeding from the nose. When abroad he had frequent attacks of catarrh; his liability to which is thought to have prevented him from settling in London, a measure which, as I have said, Mr. Hunter countenanced; but at the same time owing to his delicate health advised a return home. This liability continued with him through life—a damp floor, a slight current of air, an easterly wind, exposure to night air—almost any departure from ordinary temperature produced it, and sometimes very violently: he therefore observed a degree of precaution, which to some persons appeared as mere nervousness or affectation. I knew him intimately since the death of his nephew, Dr. Dorsey, in 1819, and may say that he never passed a day without some sensation of pain, feebleness, and derangement in his system—sometimes a catarrh—at other times a headache—sometimes pains in his kidneys with sabulous discharge—sometimes dyspepsia—at other times anasarcous swelling of the legs—and always a small, feeble, wiry pulse, irregular, and indicative of ossification, or some other change about the left valves of the heart. To these were added frequent exasperations of his habitual disorders—catarrh and nephritis—amounting to threatening illness, and from which he recovered very slowly.

For several years his debility was so great, that when the business of the day was over he had to lie down for mere animal repose, and his common hour for retiring to bed was 9 o'clock. In his intervals of better health he was up at from 6 to 7 o'clock, a.m.—he then arranged the business of the day, got his breakfast early, and went out at 8 o'clock in summer and at 9 o'clock in winter. He returned home about 1 o'clock, got his dinner, and attended to consultations in his office from 2 to 3 o'clock, p.m. His health permitting he went out again at the latter hour, and continued to make visits till sunset: he very rarely did so after sunset, or in the night, as his liability to catarrh forbade such exposure. His great enjoyment was heat: in the winter he kept his bed-room at from 75 to 80°.

During Dr. Physick's last years, Dr. Horner noted that his health "became so bad that he was accessible to few persons except his family". *By chance, Dr. Horner encountered Dr. Physick in the street on November 26, 1837.* "By this time, Dr. Physick's breathing was frequently extremely difficult, and as the anasarcous state of his legs augmented, this difficulty also increased; to assuage it he spent much of his time day and night, supported on the middle of the floor in an erect position." *In his obituary, Dr. Horner recounted their brief conversation in which Dr. Physick acknowledged his friendship and esteem for Dr. Horner while stating that,* "... I must die soon, my fate is fixed...". *The prophecy was fulfilled 19 days later on December 15, 1837. In Dr. Horner's opinion,* "The immediate cause of death was probably, from the symptoms, hydrothorax."

So protracted an illness, attended with such suffering, impaired also the vigor and clearness of his mind, and exhibited it not infrequently in strong contrast with its natural traits. He left a paper directing the disposition of his body after death, as follows: a dissection was absolutely prohibited; no one was to touch him but two females who had been his domestics, for the last twenty years. He was not to be taken from his bed for some time, but to be wrapped up in it warmly; the room was to be kept well warmed till putrefaction commenced. He was then to be covered with flannel, and placed in a wooden coffin, painted outside, with a mattress at the bottom; and this coffin was to be placed within a leaden one, and it soldered up closely. A public notice was to be given of the period of his interment, but no invitations issued.

Among the peculiar arrangements attending his death, was a rigid watch being kept for six weeks during the night over the place of his interment, and which was said to be according to his directions, to prevent the body from being disturbed. ...It, with his prohibition against the examination of his body after death, may be considered as among the sentiments incompatible with his career of surgery and anatomy, and which we can only explain by that sensitiveness, we may perhaps say obliquity, produced by long-continued retirement and indisposition.

An alternative explanation may have been Dr. Physick's desire to shield his grotesquely wasted body from the sight of the public. The corpse was described as follows by Dr. Horner:

His countenance had then a superannuated, painful, haggard expression, wrapped in the dullness and mystery of death. His frame declared his recent sufferings and exhaustion; the upper parts attenuated to a mere skeleton, the lower extremities and abdomen bloated ready to burst with dropsy, and actually beginning a sphacelated softening and ulceration, here and there. He remained a wreck merely of a divine original. *Hei mihi qualis erat, quantum mutatus.* What a contrast to that luminous and searching eye, to that countenance of thoughtful and profound reflection, to that dignity of demeanor, such as I had formerly known in him!

Earlier in the obituary, Dr. Horner had provided written snapshots of Dr. Physick's appearance that were in sharp contrast to the lugubrious post-mortem image. The living Dr. Physick had been described as follows:

Dr. Physick was of middling stature, and not inclined to corpulence even at his best periods of health. His bust was a remarkably fine one; he had a well formed head and face, the expression of the latter being thoughtful and pensive, sometimes enlivened in conversation by a smile, but very seldom so, spontaneously. His nose was aquiline and thin; and his eye hazel, well formed, vivid, and searching,—his gaze seemed sometimes to penetrate into the very interior of the body. His eye acquired additional effect from his pallid, fixed, and statue-like face. His ear was large, flat, and unhandsome, being generally concealed by the way in which he wore his hair. His hands were small, delicate, and flexible. He was not well formed in the legs and feet, the latter being rather large and flat. He dressed with great neatness; his clothes being put on with an exact attention to the process, and being from year to year of a uniform cut: blue with metal buttons was the favourite colour for his coat, a light waistcoat, and light grey or drab pantaloons.

Everyone acquainted with him must remember the neatness and conformity, one day with another, of the bow-knot in his cravat; the cleanness with which he shaved; his smooth, polished, and semi-transparent visage; the method with which every hair of his eyebrows and head had its place. The hair of the head was combed backwards from his forehead, so as to expose the entire volume of the latter. Many no doubt remember the very admirable and characteristic appearance imparted to his physiognomy and head by the use of hair powder, and how this almost solitary remnant among the gentlemen of Philadelphia of an ancient fashion, seemed to be in entire harmony with his own individuality of mind and of reputation. There are also perhaps some among us who felt a twinge of regret when, ten or twelve years ago, from sheer modesty and a desire to avoid any peculiarity of dress, he gave up this ornament, so appropriate to himself, and exposed the traces of time by the mixed hues of his locks. The queue, now so utterly exploded, he however continued to the last, but much reduced in magnitude by the successive encroachments of the scissors, and by the losses of age: this only relic of his person it is my fortune to possess.

Now as he looked at his dead friend Dr. Horner recalled his memory of Dr. Physick at the time they both attended the funeral of Dr. Benjamin Rush in 1813:

He *[Physick]* was then in the vigor of manhood and of reputation, the universally acknowledged centre and head of the surgery of this country. An indescribable interval separated him from everybody else, and yet attracted everyone to him. I remember with perfect distinctness, as he turned off from the ground, his quick and thoughtful step; his inclination of the head: as either musing on what he had seen, or ruminating on some case of profound interest then under his charge. His appearance such as in his most palmy days—his head highly powdered; his hair overhanging his ears in a thick long brush on each side, where it was clipped straight below. The head, face, and neck, exhibiting the most finished and statue-like appearance; and his costume being a paragon of neatness, and of appropriateness, without any undue effort at effect. I never saw him before or since more completely himself. The attack of typhus-fever, which he had the next winter, altered sensibly for the remainder of his life, the face—the forehead never recovered its fullness.

Dr. Physick's desire to shield his grotesquely wasted body from the sight of the public may have reflected his recognition that he had once been perceived as "a beautiful man" and ageless. He managed to maintain this image all the way out to 1831, with the aid of his most successful surgical case.

His operation for the stone on Chief Justice Marshall, in 1831, was the last of his great efforts. He anticipated it with much anxiety, but when brought to the point he rallied finely—everything was as usual in readiness. The unexpected turn given to the operation, by the almost incredible number, probably a thousand small calculi which he met with, and their adhesion to the internal coat of the bladder, did not disconcert him in the slightest degree. He in a little time detected the existing state of things, and they were brought to a successful conclusion, being followed by a complete cure. This operation was the more interesting from the distinction of its two principal personages; the one, the acknowledged head of the legal profession, and the other of the medical: and both sustaining themselves; though in advanced life, by that tone of moral firmness and dignity which had advanced them from inconsiderable beginnings, to the stations which they then occupied.

After turning the anatomy Chair over to his successor, Dr. Horner in 1831, Dr. Physick still had 6 more years to live.

Some of the incidents of the doctor's last sickness, marking the decrepitude into which he had fallen, transpired, so as to become the subjects of public conversation: for to him was not granted the boon so eloquently expressed in the message of the Senate to the President of the United States, on the death of General Washington; that "Favoured of Heaven, he departed without exhibiting the weakness of humanity." Surely to the intelligent no apology can be wanting for the infirmities of age and of illness, and yet it is but too true that the public sensibilities were moved. Can it be peculiar to our city that she is fastidious about her great men? That she is better pleased when they die like demigods in the midst of their glory? …She certainly feels impatient and excited when she hears that they have undergone the common lot of declining humanity; that the pains, the capriciousness, the imbecilities of mind and body of old age, have also come upon them…Philadelphia requires that the ermine of reputation be neither stained, torn, nor abused in any way; that the character itself should correspond with the hypothetical perfection and greatness which are presumed to attend it: and she denies to age its great privilege of returning once more to childhood.

All of his responsible public appointments, excepting that of the presidency of the Medical Society, had been resigned; and the only connection which he then held with the University of Pennsylvania, was in the titular honor of Emeritus Professor of Surgery and Anatomy, conferred upon him in 1831, upon his vacating the latter chair. The solitary duty connected with the appointment was that of signing the diplomas; but even this duty became so irksome to him that for the last two years he had declined it.

Dr. Physick's legacy had, in fact, long since outgrown Philadelphia. Dr. Horner's list of Dr. Physick's achievements began with Physick's public health measures to control yellow fever: i.e. the peoples' responsibility for … "cleanliness at their own doors and along their own wharves"…To this idea, constantly urged upon public attention, we owe the very complete and effective arrangement for supplying this city with water…

To the walks of surgery, however, we must look for the genius of Physick in its most decided and extensive application. It is there that we find it exhibiting a series of triumphs, over cases of disease which had baffled the skill of men only inferior to himself, and it is there that it was so active in inventions, to improve and to palliate established modes of treatment. His management of diseased joints by perfect rest, elevation, and diet, is a happy substitute for the errors generated under the use of the terms scrofula—white swelling: and ending either by amputation or in death, sometimes in both. His treatment of the inflammation of the hip-joint in children (coxalgia), by a splint, low diet, and frequent purging, exhibits another of those successful innovations upon ordinary practice. His invention of an appropriate treatment and cure for that loathsome disease artificial anus, which invention has been so unceremoniously modified and claimed by a distinguished French surgeon, the late Baron Dupuytren, is a proof of the activity and resources of his professional mind. Another invention still more frequent in its employment, from the greater number of such cases, is the application of the seton to the cure of fractures of bones refusing to unite.

Other inventions are found in the treatment of mortification by blisters; of anthrax by caustic alkali; of the ligature of kid skin for arteries, in excisions of the female breast. To him also we owe the original act, if not invention, of pumping out the stomach in cases of poisoning: also an improvement in the treatment of fractures of the condyles of the os humeri, so as to render the restoration perfect. I might in this way go on to enumerate many other points of excellence about him, but however appropriate it might be to offer a complete exposition of them, the time allotted to a ceremonial of this kind must prohibit a more extensive and complete annunciation. Those who have had an opportunity of witnessing his practice extensively will at least conclude with me in the saying, *Nihil tetigit, quod non ornavit*.

With this great fertility in invention and ardour in the prosecution of his profession, his original papers are deplorably few, and they are also very short. I doubt whether they exceed much half a dozen in number, and whether thirty or forty pages printed in common type would not contain all. Lecturing for many years on surgery, his chief organ of publicity was his class of students. The Elements of Surgery, published by his nephew, Dr. Dorsey, contain the most perfect account of his opinions and practice up to that period: The Institutes and Practice of Surgery, by Dr. Gibson, the present able and distinguished professor of surgery in the University of Pennsylvania, represents largely his views obtained through private communication and publications. Other individuals have also been, through their writings, the means of his intercourse with the press on particular points; among them may be mentioned Dr. J. Randolph, his son-in-law; Drs. Benjamin and Reynell Coates; and, to some degree, myself. Whether these several sources of information, do not furnish nearly all of an original kind which he himself would have advanced, may remain unsettled as a question; but my opinion is, that nearly the whole fund is supplied. This however I say with great regret at his reserve as a writer. Lamentations of the same kind have been made in the case of Dessault, for it is almost entirely through his pupils that his reputation is transmitted. I may perhaps be pardoned for the allusion, in saying, that in an instance of unequalled importance, the foundation of Christianity, we have no original document, it is all through disciples.

To the preceding claims to our professional veneration, were united physical qualifications of the most perfect kind. He had a correct, sharp, discriminating eye; a hand delicate in its touch and movement, and which never trembled or faltered; an entire composure, and self-possession, the energy of which increased upon an unexpected emergency. He had a forethought of all possible contingencies and demands during a great operation, and therefore had everything prepared for it; when performed he entered upon a most conscientious discharge of his duty to the patient, and watched him with a vigilance and anxiety which never remitted till his fate was ascertained. If to the foregoing brilliant qualities as an operator, and the loud plaudits which attended their exercise, we add a chastening of feeling, which subdued every sentiment of vanity, and regulated entirely his judgment; and that he had an invincible repugnance, a horror at engaging in dangerous operations through ostentation, and where the probabilities of cure were not largely in favour of the patient: we have in this summary the most perfect example of a surgeon, which this country has ever seen. But as these great points and striking professional land-marks seldom come in clusters, it will probably be long in the course of Providence before there will be a reunion of all the same qualities.

In Dr. Horner's view, fame and fortune did not bring to Dr. Physick an ease of mind. Religion did not help.

The doctrines of theology occupied much of his attention for twenty years or more before he died; yet it must be admitted that he derived a very doubtful satisfaction from them. Its dogmatic points were always the subjects of inquietude, and never fully received by him; difficulties great and small were constantly present to his imagination. His profession made him the witness of so much human pain and misery, that he did not know how to reconcile it with what was said of the goodness of the Creator… . His sombre and questionable view of the benevolence of the Deity, no doubt arose from his bad state of health excluding him from everything like personal enjoyment, or a deliberate survey of the glories and beauties, I may say beatitudes of nature; and from his mind being therefore never relieved from its achings produced, by his routine of professional duty.

The "age of enlightenment" in which the rise of science and "philosophy" were handmaidens also failed to bring comfort.

Philosophy certainly has its trials. In forming the mind to the interrogation of the visible world : in expanding its powers, and in assimilating it to beings of unearthly existence, it creates while we are in health and sound, a confidence of ourselves and in our own powers, which makes us believe that we are equal to any possible state of things. But let us turn from this buoyant and exhilarated state, and imagine ourselves in the solitude and pain of a sick chamber, with the conviction that death is advancing with an unfailing and steady step: where is that process of chemical analysis or of logical deduction, which enlightens us in regard to its character, and braces the nerves for the meeting? … where is that dissection of the heart, of the brain, or of any other part, which has revealed the grand mystery? All knowledge is emptiness itself, or a misty vision… . How strangely does the inside of a great man contrast with the outside—with the part and the appendages that the world sees, and delusively believes to be the source of unfailing happiness.

On his demise, testimonies of respect for his memory were adopted at many distant places, in the form of resolutions from medical bodies… . It is not a little remarkable in these and other expressions of public opinion, that in the bodies represented (acting as they did without concert or knowledge of each other's proceedings) the term, " Father of American Surgery," heretofore much in use, has been almost universally adopted; so that it may now be considered as irrevocably fixed, under that rule of theology which admits as incontrovertible *"quod semper et ubique et ab omnibus"*. We therefore now hail him again in this place under the Title of Father of American Surgery, and let no hand at any future day be so presumptuous, or so arrogant, as to attempt to tear down this honourable inscription to his memory.

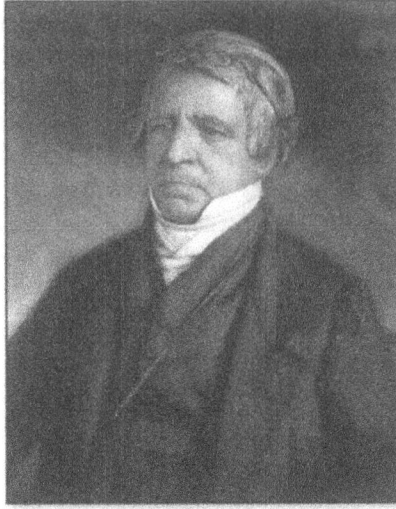

NATHANIEL CHAPMAN

1780–1853 (APS 1807)

Memoir by John B. Biddle

Nathaniel Chapman, ninth President of the American Philosophical Society, was descended from an ancient and honorable English family. His paternal ancestor came to Virginia with the very first colony, under the auspices of Raleigh, to whom he was nearly related by blood. He had been a captain of cavalry in the British army, and received a considerable grant of land in the new territory, upon which his distinguished kinsman had just bestowed the appellation of the Virgin Queen.

The old seat of the Chapman family in Virginia is still in their possession, on the river Pomonkey, some twenty miles above Richmond. A branch of the family, about the year 1700, migrated to the adjoining State of Maryland, and fixed itself on the banks of the Potomac, nearly opposite Mount Vernon. They retained the designation of the ancient settlement, and called the new estate Pomonkey. From this branch Dr. Chapman is descended. His father, however, returned to Virginia upon his marriage, and passed his life there. His wife was of that Scotch stock, of which so many were attracted to Virginia, in the early days of her tobacco trade. She was the daughter of Allan Macrae, of Dumfries, in Virginia, a merchant and tobacco factor, who accumulated a large fortune, which he bequeathed to his children.

Nathaniel Chapman, the second son of George Chapman and Amelia Macrae, was born on the 18th May, 1780, at his father's seat, Summer Hill, in Fairfax County, Virginia, on the banks of the Potomac. The ancient town of Alexandria, then the capital of northeastern Virginia, was within a few miles of the seat of the Chapmans; and about equidistant stood the future site of Washington.

At a very early age Chapman commenced the study of the profession which he so long illustrated and adorned. In the year 1797, when but little more than seventeen years of age, he came up to

Philadelphia, for attendance on the medical lectures at the University of Pennsylvania. For two years previously he had been engaged in a course of preliminary reading, under the guidance of two neighboring physicians, both in their day men of no little note. A year he spent in the office of Dr. John Weems, of Georgetown, afterwards and now of the District of Columbia. Weems, a close friend and near relation of the Chapman family, was a practitioner of much local eminence. From his office, Chapman passed under the care of Dr. Dick, of Alexandria, then and still favorably known in the annals of American medicine.

At seventeen, a stranger, without fortune, connections, or influence, Chapman launched his bark in the crowded metropolis of the United States. At thirty-three, he had reached the front rank of his profession. Seated in a leading chair of the renowned American school of medicine, with the most desirable practice of a great city at his command, an eminent social favorite, distinguished as a wit and conversationalist, he enjoyed a position which left him nothing to desire.

Upon his arrival in Philadelphia, Chapman became the private pupil of Rush, then in the zenith of his popularity and influence. With Rush he soon made himself a favorite, and there is little doubt that he was early destined by his preceptor for introduction into the University, if not for the succession to the Chair of Practice. The Medical Faculty of the University of Pennsylvania, in the days of Chapman's pupilage, presented an array of names, which, with scarcely an exception, have become historical. Shippen, Wistar, Rush, Barton, and Woodhouse, filled the four chairs, to which the organization was limited.

Upon his graduation in the spring of 1800, Chapman presented an inaugural thesis on Hydrophobia, written at the request of Rush, in an answer to an attack on the Professor's favorite theory of the pathology of that disease. He had previously prepared an essay on the sympathetic connections of the stomach with the rest of the body. This paper, afterwards read before the Philadelphia Medical Society, contained the germs of Chapman's doctrines, regarding the pathology of fever, as well as the modus operandi of medicines.

Chapman did not obtain the advantage of an hospital residence, upon his graduation. But Chapman, destitute of influence in these quarters, determined to seek the most celebrated schools and hospitals of Europe, with the view to the completion of his medical education. He remained abroad three years, nearly one of which he spent in London, a private pupil of Abernethy's. This celebrated man had great powers as a teacher, and an unrivalled faculty of impressing the minds of his students. The founder of the Physiological School of Surgery, and the author of a rational constitutional treatment of surgical diseases, he carried his pathological views also into the domain of Medicine.

Constitutional disorders, he maintained, either originate from, or are allied with derangements of the stomach and bowels, and can be reached only through these organs. These doctrines probably took no little hold of the mind of his young American pupil. They are traceable throughout his future teachings and writings. There was something, moreover, congenial in the temperaments of the two men; but Chapman had Abernethy's humor, without a tinge of his coarseness and causticity.

Edinburgh, however, was at this time the medical metropolis of the world; and, in 1801, Chapman went there for a sojourn of two years. The influences which the Edinburgh medical school had long exerted over the profession of America is forcibly described by Dr. Jackson in his Discourse commemorative of Dr. Chapman. "The celebrity it had acquired from its Monroe, Cullen, Brown, and Gregory, had not been eclipsed by the Paris or German schools, or rivalled by those of London or Dublin. The medical school of the Scotch metropolis was the cynosure of American physicians during the colonial period, and continued to be so until within the last twenty-five years. Most of the eminent medical men of Philadelphia, New York, and Boston, of the latter part of the last century, were its alumni. I doubt whether, at that time, more was known of the European continental schools than the mere existence of two or three of repute. All of the medical doctrines, ideas, principles, and practice of this country were derived from the Edinburgh school, or from English writers.

The great ornament of the Edinburgh school, Cullen, had been, at this time, some years dead. But his teachings survived, and, indeed, pervaded not only the British isles, but the North American continent. The doctrines of Cullen, which are to a certain extent founded upon those of Hoffman, had effected a revolution in medical theories. They superseded the humoral pathology of Boerhaave, and based diseased action solely upon derangement of the solid organs of the body. The system of Cullen, afterwards rudely simplified by Brown, and again modified by Rush, retained its hold over the British and American mens medica, until the comparatively recent discoveries of chemical analysis revived the old humoral opinions, so consonant with the instincts of mankind. Chapman carried away with him for life the doctrines of the Edinburgh school. He was, to the close of his medical career, in the language of Dr. Jackson, "a most uncompromising vitalist and solidist."

His residence in Edinburgh was agreeable as well as instructive. His pleasant manners and social powers brought him into intimacy with a number of distinguished men, particularly Lord Buchan, Dugald Stewart, and Brougham. He seems to have anticipated the career of Brougham; for, not long after his return to the United States, he republished Brougham's speech before the House of Commons on the British Orders in Council, with a biographical sketch, in which the eminence of the future chancellor was predicted.

Lord Buchan, the eccentric but warm-hearted friend of America and Americans, paid the young Virginian the compliment of a public breakfast, upon his departure for his own country. The occasion selected was the birthday of Washington, and a large number of distinguished persons, including most of the literary celebrities of the modern Athens and many of the nobility, male and female, were present. Lord Buchan, at the close of this entertainment, committed to the custody of his young friend an interesting relic, valuable from a double historical association. He had, some years previously, presented to General Washington a box made from the oak that sheltered Wallace after the battle of Falkirk, with a request to pass it at his death to the man in his country who should appear to merit it best. General Washington, declining so invidious a designation, returned it by will to the Earl, who intrusted it to Dr. Chapman, with a view to its being ultimately placed in the cabinet of the College at Washington, to which General Washington had made a bequest.

Upon his return to the United States, Chapman determined to select Philadelphia as the theatre of his professional career, and in 1804 commenced the labors of his profession in Philadelphia. His success was immediate; and for a period of nearly fifty years he commanded whatever he could attend of practice in the most refined and opulent circles of our city.

As a practitioner, his qualifications were unrivalled. The charm of his manner was no less effective in the sick-chamber than his skill in distinguishing and relieving disease. His lively conversation and ever-ready joke were often more soothing than anodyne or cordial; and when roused by urgent symptoms, he was unequalled in resources, as he was devoted in attentions. As a consulting physician, his great powers were particularly conspicuous. Rapid and clear in diagnosis, inexhaustible in therapeutics, self-relying, never discouraged, never "giving up the ship," he was the physician of physicians for an emergency. At the bedside, Chapman dismissed speculative theories of morbid action. His remedies were drawn from observation and experience; and no man wielded more dexterously and successfully the known resources of his time. In our day, a less depressing therapeutics has come into fashion, and the means of combating disease are doubtless more numerous than they were in Chapman's hands. But, "Take him for all in all, We shall not look upon his like again."

He was singularly indifferent to the emoluments of his profession. Careless in his accounts, resolute in refusing bills to his numerous family connections and personal friends, always moderate in his charges, he realized scarcely a tithe of the receipts which some of his successors in fashionable practice have rolled up. No more generous and less covetous man ever lived.

Public teaching early attracted Chapman's aspirations. Very soon after his return from Europe he gave a private course on Obstetrics, a branch which had then merely a nominal place in the lectures at the University. His success led, in 1807–8, to a connection with James, already known as a teacher of obstetrics. In 1810, the Professorship of Midwifery in the University was conferred upon James, with an understanding that he should be assisted by Chapman. His introduction into the University was now fixed; but an independent chair was not placed within his reach until, in 1813, the death of Rush occasioned a rearrangement of the school. Barton, who had long filled the chair of Materia Medica with distinguished eclat, was induced to exchange it for that of the theory and Practice; and the former chair, thus made vacant, was conferred upon Chapman.

During the brief period in which Chapman occupied the chair of Materia Medica, his courses were eminently satisfactory to his classes. Dr. Jackson considers them "an advance on those of his predecessor," and Caldwell bears strong testimony to his success. His lectures were afterwards embodied in his "Elements of Therapeutics and Materia Medica," a work justly pronounced by Dr. Jackson to have been "the best treatise in the English language on those subjects at the time of its publication."

Chapman's Therapeutics is an original work—original in its plan, original in its execution. As a text-book, it is of course superseded by later publications; but the American student will do well not to "lay it on the shelf." The chapter on Emetics will never be obsolete. The solidist doctrines of the day were adopted by Chapman in explanation of the modus operandi of medicines. Their absorption into the blood had scarcely yet been demonstrated by physiology; and the principle of SYMPATHY, which he employed to account for morbid action, he applied also to the explanation of medicinal impressions. But, with singular candor, when Magendie's experiments on the absorption of medicines were announced, Chapman "engaged Drs. Coates, Lawrence, and Harlan, to repeat them at his expense;" and, upon their confirmation, although he made no public recantation of his views, he would never permit the publication of another edition of his work. It had already gone through seven editions, one of them surreptitious; and "when still in great demand, the author refused to have it reprinted, because he thought it required a thorough revision."

The great event of Chapman's life was his appointment, in 1816, to the Chair of the Theory and Practice of Medicine and Clinical Medicine, in the University of Pennsylvania. He filled it for more than a third of a century, with distinguished success; and left it with a national reputation. His lectures were enriched with varied erudition; in style forcible and terse. His medical opinions, accordant in the main with the approved dogma of his time, were in much original. His practical precepts were judicious and impressive.

As a lecturer, he is well portrayed by his colleague, Dr. Jackson, "as self-possessed, deliberate, and empathic. Whenever warmed with his subject, his animation became oratorical. Often the tedium of dry matter would be enlivened by some stroke of wit, a happy pun, an anecdote, or quotation. He was furnished with stores of facts and cases, drawn from his own large experience and observation, illustrating principles, disease, or treatment, under discussion. His bearing was dignified, his manner was easy and his gestures were graceful. He had a thorough command over the attention of his class, with whom he always possessed an unbounded popularity. His voice had a peculiar intonation, depending on some defect in the confirmation of the palate, that rendered the articulation of certain sounds an effort. The first time he was heard, the ear experienced difficulty in distinguishing his words. This was of short duration; for once accustomed to the tone, his enunciation was remarkable for its distinctness. Students would often take notes of his lectures nearly verbatim."

Chapman's leading Theory of Medicine was comprised in the great principle, SYMPATHY. His predecessor, Rush, refining on the solidism of the Scotch school, had reduced all diseases to a unit,— considering them to be mere expressions of different states of excitability and degrees of excitement. Chapman "recognized the differences in the vital endowments of the tissues and organs, and the diversities of pathological conditions." He restored the classification of diseases which Rush had discarded. Adopting the prevailing anti-humoral views, he refused, however, to deny the obvious and well-defined varieties in the manifestations of disease; and skilfully expanded his theories to include them.

In the spring of 1850, the decline of health and physical powers led Dr. Chapman to abandon the field of labor which he had so long and brilliantly occupied. He resigned his chair, and withdrew from practice and society. For three years, he survived, in the seclusion of his family; slowly and almost imperceptibly, without apparent disease, by gentle and gradual decay, passing to the other world. His death took place on the 1st of July, 1853.

The highest complimentary distinctions, which his professional brethren could accord, had been paid Dr. Chapman, He was for many years President of the Philadelphia Medical Society; and was by acclamation, in 1848, elected first President of the American Medical Association. Many medical and learned societies of Europe also enrolled him among their members. In 1846, he was elected to the Presidency of the Society. He held it three years, declining a re-election in 1849.

Chapman's personal popularity was not inferior to his professional position. His temperament was cast in the happiest mould. Social in disposition, with an unfailing gaiety of spirit, a wit—a punster—delightful as a companion, and enjoying company, he, for a generation, occupied a position unrivaled in the society of Philadelphia. To these brilliant qualities, he united the kindliest feelings and the gentlest temper. He was utterly without malice; frank, open-hearted, and open-handed. His jokes and puns are familiar in our Philadelphia ears as household words; and those who enjoyed the charm of his society will not soon forget his cordial, blithesome manner, and his bright, cheery look.

Dr. Chapman's published writings are numerous. His "Therapeutics" has been alluded to. Many of his lectures appeared in the "Medical Examiner" of Philadelphia, in the years 1838, 1839, and 1840, and were afterwards republished, with others, in separate form. The published lectures comprise the following subjects, viz.: Eruptive Fevers, Diseases of the Thoracic Viscera, Fevers, Dropsy, Gout, and Rheumatism. A compendium of his Lectures was also published by Dr. N.D. Benedict. In 1820, Dr. Chapman commenced the publication of *The Philadelphia Journal of the Medical and Physical Sciences*, which he continued to edit for many years. This Journal, continued to the present day, under the name of *The American Journal of the Medical Sciences*, is now well known throughout Europe and America as the oldest and first of American medical journals.

In 1804, Dr. Chapman contracted a matrimonial alliance, from which he derived unalloyed happiness. His wife, Rebecca Biddle (daughter of Colonel Clement Biddle, of the Revolutionary Army, an intimate friend and confidential correspondent of Washington's), still survives him.

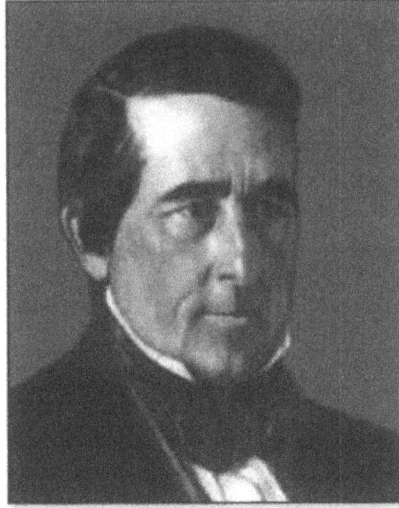

FRANKLIN BACHE

1792–1864 (APS 1820)
Memoir by George Bacon Wood

The members of the American Philosophical Society need not to be informed that Dr. Bache was the great-grandson of its founder and first President, Dr. Benjamin Franklin. Sarah, Dr. Franklin's only daughter, was married to Richard Bache, an English gentleman, who emigrated, when a young man, to this country, from near Preston, in Lancashire, and became a citizen of Pennsylvania. The eldest child of this marriage, Benjamin Franklin Bache, was the father of our deceased fellow-member, who was born in Philadelphia on the 25th of October, 1792, and, in consequence of the early death of his father, was, with several younger brothers, left to the care of their mother, aided, for a considerable portion of their minority, by her second husband, William Duane.

The early education of Dr. Bache was similar to that of most other youths destined for a liberal profession. He graduated in the department of arts of the University of Pennsylvania in 1810, and entering immediately on the study of medicine, went through a regular course of instruction, and received the degree of doctor of medicine in the medical department of the same school in 1814. In the preceding year, he had been appointed surgeon's mate in the army, and in the course of service, after his graduation, became surgeon; a position which he continued to hold until the then existing war with Great Britain closed, and for a short time subsequently. In 1816, however, he resigned, in order to engage in the practice of his profession in Philadelphia.

Dr. Bache exhibited a very early predilection for chemistry. Soon after commencing his medical studies, in the year 1811, he published, in the Aurora newspaper, an essay on the probable composition of muriatic acid, a question which long agitated the scientific world, and which, even after the discovery of chlorine, remained for many years unsettled. Dr. Bache seems to have been an early convert from the old hypothesis, which regarded chlorine as a compound of muriatic acid and oxygen, and the acid as yet undecomposed, to the new doctrine of Sir Humphry Davy, which taught that chlorine was simple, and muriatic acid a compound of it and hydrogen.

Until the discovery of iodine and bromine, the close analogy of which with chlorine rendered infinitely probable a similar analogy in their relations with other bodies, no experimentum crucis had been made sufficient to satisfy all minds of the truth of the elementary doctrine; and it is a singular fact, that, in the almost countless ramifications into which the inquiry was pushed, explanation was in every instance possible as well upon the one as upon the other of these so different and even contradictory hypotheses. There are very few coincidences so remarkable in the whole history of the science.

In 1813, before his graduation in medicine, Dr. Bache published three chemical papers in the "Memoirs of the Columbian Chemical Society." He appears to have suspended his chemical studies upon entering the army, and not to have resumed them until after his return to Philadelphia, in 1816. But he must then have recommenced them with great ardor; for near the close of 1819, appeared his "System of Chemistry for the Use of Students of Medicine," an elementary treatise in one octavo volume of somewhat more than six hundred pages. This work was based upon Dr. Thompson's treatise, but contains much material industriously gathered from other sources, and, in its arrangement and execution, evinces so many of the characteristic traits of the author as fully to justify its claims to originality. Method, precision, accuracy, and simplicity, are its prominent features; and thus, with the very great modification and vast expansion which chemistry has undergone since it made its appearance, the book, without very material changes, would not meet the present wants of the student, it was, nevertheless, when published, a good epitome of the science.

In 1821, in conjunction with Dr. Hare, he edited the first American edition of Ure's Dictionary of Chemistry; in 1823, prepared a supplementary volume to Henry's Chemistry, republished by Robert Desilver; in 1825, edited anonymously "A System of Pyrotechny," written by Dr. James Cutbush, of the United States Army, who died just as he had completed the manuscript; and in 1830, contributed to the "Philadelphia Journal of Health," an article on purifying and disinfecting agents, and edited the third edition of Turner's Chemistry. The last-mentioned work was an excellent elementary treatise, and exceedingly popular in the United States as long as the author lived. Dr. Bache edited four successive American editions; and there can be no doubt that he contributed much to its general acceptance in this country, by his most careful and conscientious revisions.

From chemical authorship the attention of Dr. Bache was naturally turned to chemical teaching, and he began to lecture on the subject as early as 1821. Probably, in order to test his capacity before entering on a larger field, he made his first attempt in the presence of a class consisting exclusively of his brothers, sisters, and other near relatives; but soon afterwards he lectured to the private medical students of his friend, Dr. Thomas T. Hewson, and still later to a much larger class, composed of the joint pupils of two private summer medical schools, at that time established in Philadelphia.

While thus teaching medical classes in the summer, he delivered, also, courses in the winter, first to the pupils of the Franklin Institute, in which he became Professor of Chemistry in 1826, and afterwards to classes of pharmaceutical students in the Philadelphia College of Pharmacy, by which he was appointed to the same professorship in the year 1831.

While thus engaged in teaching chemistry, both as a writer and lecturer, he did not neglect his professional business. To his private practice, which came very slowly, and never in a degree equivalent to his merits, were added, for several years, the official duties of inspecting recruits for the United States army, and of attending military officers who might happen to require medical aid when stationed in Philadelphia. He was, moreover, for a considerable time, physician both to the old Walnut Street Prison and to the new Penitentiary at Cherry Hill, to the former of which he was appointed in 1824, and to the latter in 1829.

Besides these avocations, which yielded him more or less income, he was for a period of six years, from 1826 to 1832, engaged, with several others, in gratuitously conducting the North American Medical and Surgical Journal, one of the best medical periodicals then existing, which occupied much of his time and thoughts; and in the year 1829, he entered upon another course of unpaid labor, on the part of the College of Physicians of this city, in revising the United States Pharmacopoeia, which was repeated every ten years as long as he lived.

In the year 1818, soon after having established himself as a practitioner of medicine in Philadelphia, Dr. Bache married Aglae, the daughter of Jean Dabadie, a French gentleman then resident in this city. Perhaps by the merely worldly-wise this may have been regarded as an imprudent step, as their united incomes were insufficient for the support of a family; and for many years, with all that he could add to that income by his best exertions, the young couple labored under many difficulties from deficient means, which were, of course, aggravated by the constantly increasing family that was growing up around them. Nevertheless, I have no doubt that he acted most wisely; for the match was one of affection; the lady was intelligent, amiable, and in every way worthy of him.

Unhappily, Mrs. Bache, after bearing with her husband the difficulties of his earlier career, was called away from him just as his pecuniary affairs were beginning to be no longer a source of anxiety. She died of consumption in May, 1835, leaving him, as her best legacy, a young family of sons and daughters to give exercise to his affections, and comfort to his declining years.

I shall treat first of his relations with this Society, with which he was so long and so intimately associated. He was elected a member on the 1st of April, 1822. For several years there is little evidence, in the minutes of the Society, that he participated actively in its proceedings otherwise than by attendance at its meetings; the only office filled by him previously to the year 1825 being that of judge of the annual election in January, 1822.

He was too modest to draw attention to himself by any premature display; so that, in looking over the records, I have noticed only a single instance, during the first five years of his membership, in which he appears to have departed from his rule of silence; and, in this instance, it was nothing of his own that he offered, but a paper by Mr. Henry Seibert, containing the results of an analysis of a specimen of fluosilicate of magnesia from New Jersey.

In the regularity of his attendance he was very remarkable, from the date of his election to that of his decease; and certainly, during this long period, there was no other member of the Society who was present at nearly so many meetings as he. A record of attendance has been kept by the Treasurer since the beginning of 1850; and from that year, inclusive, to 1864, which was the last of Dr. Bache's life, his average yearly attendance, notwithstanding an absence from the country on one occasion of five or six months, was fifteen meetings, the whole annual number being twenty. The only other member who, during this period, exhibited so fair a record, or even an approach to it, was our worthy Treasurer himself, whose favorable line of marks for most of the time was almost without a flaw.

In January, 1825, Dr. Bache was elected one of the Secretaries, and he continued to serve the Society faithfully in this capacity until January, 1843, having been the senior Secretary for eleven years. For a considerable portion of the same time he was one of the Standing Committee of Publication, having been appointed a member of the Committee in 1826, and its chairman in 1829; and he continued to act in the latter capacity until January 1835, when he declined a reappointment.

At the election of January 1843, he was chosen one of the Vice-Presidents of the Society, and, being re-elected annually, became senior Vice-President in 1849. This relative position he continued to hold until January, 1853, when, Dr. R. M. Patterson having on account of his failing health declined a re-election, he was chosen President; thus having risen regularly through successive grade of office to the highest, as if the Society, in its relations with him, had participated in that spirit of order by which he was himself so strongly characterized.

During the first year of his presidency, he paid, with myself, a visit of five or six months to Europe. On this occasion the Society furnished him with a circular to its correspondents abroad, which facilitated his intercourse with scientific men, and would have been still more useful, had not the necessary rapidity of our movements very much curtailed his opportunities for such intercourse. But throughout the journey he kept the good of the Society in view, searching for information about its foreign members, endeavoring to awaken an interest in its affairs among those he was happy enough to meet, and seeking to extend its relations, both with individuals and associations, whenever apparently desirable.

After his return, he gave, December 16th, 1853, an address to the Society in relation to its affairs, an abstract of which is contained in the published Proceedings of that year. In consequence of a by-law then existing, "that no person should be eligible as President at more than two out of three successive elections," he ceased to hold the office after January, 1855. Believing that this rule did not work beneficially for the Society, he introduced a resolution, November 5th, 1858, after the decease of the late President, Judge Kane, for the repeal of the by-law, which at the subsequent meeting was carried by a majority of 23 to 2.

Before initiating this measure, he had firmly resolved not again to accept the responsibilities of the position; and, though the general feeling of the members was, I believe, in favor of his re-election, and he was strongly urged to permit himself to be considered as a candidate at the approaching election in January, 1859, he adhered to his resolution, and continued a private member during the residue of his life. His interest, however, in the Society, in no degree abated; and he continued to be as assiduous as ever in his attendance at the meetings, and as actively participant in the proceedings. How much the Society was present in his thoughts, may be inferred from the fact, that, on his death-bed, just before his intellect was swallowed up in stupor, he spoke to me of a measure then under the consideration of the Society, which he feared, if adopted, might prove injurious to its interests; and these were among the last intelligent words that he uttered.

In the course of his membership, Dr. Bache rendered several important services to the Society, which are worthy of being recalled. The first that I shall notice concerned the catalogue of members. Soon after he was first chosen one of the Secretaries, it was resolved, at his suggestion, that such a catalogue should be prepared by these officers; and ever afterwards he appeared to take it under his special guardianship, being always solicitous that it should be at once complete and correct, with every name properly entered, and every date, whether of the election, resignation or decease of a member, accurately stated. On the last point he often took great pains in making inquiries, especially as to the foreign members; and in regard to the subject generally, there was no one, I presume, who nearly equalled him in a careful watchfulness over the necrology of the Society, the whole number of deaths, reported by him as they became known, scarcely falling short of one hundred.

The arrangements of the Franklin papers is another result which may be fairly ascribed to him.

As they came into the possession of the Society, these papers were in a chaotic state, which rendered them almost useless for reference. In November, 1849, Dr. Bache introduced the subject to the notice of the Society; and at the following meeting in December, was made chairman of a committee, with instructions to have the papers arranged in chronological order, and divided into volumes of a convenient size for binding.

A little examination sufficed to convince the committee of the almost Herculean character of the task confided to them; and, on their recommendation, it was determined that the labor should be intrusted to some competent person, to be duly compensated. It was estimated that the papers would form at least sixty respectable folio volumes; and as ten dollars per volume was deemed but a moderate recompense for the requisite labor, the sum of six hundred dollars was appropriated to defray the cost.

The task was undertaken by our Treasurer, Mr. Trego; but so complicated and tedious did it prove, that, though he devoted to it most of the time he could spare from other avocations, it was completed only a short time before the decease of Dr. Bache. I have been told that one of the last acts of our departed friend was to appoint a meeting, with a qualified person, in order to make arrangements for the binding of these volumes; but he was prevented by his illness from fulfilling the appointment, and the work still remains to be done.

Yet another service meriting special notice was his participation in the business of newly arranging the library of the Society, and preparing a catalogue; a duty which fell to the lot of our present Librarian, and has been so well performed by him. Towards these purposes, Dr. Bache made the liberal contribution of five hundred dollars on two successive occasions, in the years 1853 and 1854, which is to be valued the more, as it proceeded not from superfluity of means, but from an income which, though considerable at the time, was all needed, in order to make prudent provision for the future of his family.

It has been already stated that, in the year 1829, Dr. Bache became engaged, with others, in the laborious duty of revising the Pharmacopoeia of the United States. He entered upon that duty as one of a committee of the College of Physicians of Philadelphia; and afterwards served on another committee appointed by the Medical Convention which met at Washington in 1830, whose duty it was to further revise and ultimately publish that important work. At three decennial periods subsequently, 1840, 1850, and 1860, he was engaged in the same manner, in the same work, and on the last of these occasions, acted as chairman of the Committee of Revision and Publication, and consequently had the chief laboring oar.

Except by the medical gentlemen present, the work here referred to can scarcely be appreciated in regard either to its importance, or the amount of labor involved; but some idea may be formed on both of these points, when it is understood that the Pharmacopoeia is a national code, essential to the maintenance throughout the country of a certain uniformity in the nomenclature and preparation of medicines, without which every member of the community would be liable to serious accidents to his health and life; and that in each revision of it, many months, and sometimes even years, are occupied with more or less work every day, to fit it for the purposes it has to fulfill. In Europe this duty is generally performed under legal sanction, and by compensated labor. With us the Pharmacopoeia rests entirely upon opinion, and all the labor bestowed and time consumed are wholly gratuitous.

Immediately after the publication of the first revised edition of the Pharmacopoeia in 1831, Dr. Bache, jointly with myself, undertook the preparation of the Dispensatory of the United States, which was completed and published in 1833. I am precluded, by my share in the authorship of that work, from treating either of its merits or demerits. This much, however, I may be permitted to say, that it purports to represent the existing state of Materia Medica and Pharmacy, has been accepted in this capacity to a great extent throughout the United States, and has been used as a guide in relation to these branches of medicine by a large proportion of the physicians and apothecaries of our country.

The extensive use of the book rendered frequent editions necessary, and thus gave opportunity for revisions at short intervals, by which its character as a representative of the knowledge of the times has been maintained. Indeed, before the decease of Dr. Bache, so many changes had been made, and so much novel matter introduced, that it had become almost a new work, possessing little more than the general features of the original. Between the years 1833, when it was first published, and 1864, when Dr. Bache died, it went through eleven editions, at average intervals of three years; having, during this time, swollen from somewhat more than a thousand to nearly sixteen hundred pages, and containing, from its greater compactness, almost twice as much matter as in the beginning.

From this statement it will be understood how great an amount of labor must have been bestowed on it from first to last by Dr. Bache, and how constant a source of occupation it must have been to him during this long period of more than thirty years. Happily the pecuniary results were such as to make his income, much restricted anteriorly to its publication, comparatively easy from that time onward, and quite adequate to his wants. The work was, moreover, a stepping-stone to his appointment to the chemical professorship in the Jefferson Medical College, which he received in 1841, and continued to hold as long as he lived.

The vicissitudes of his life seem to have ceased with this appointment. Made by it not only comfortable but even affluent in his circumstances, he was no longer compelled to search for a new and better position; and as his time and powers were sufficiently occupied in the performance of his regular duties—the care, namely, of his practice, the fulfillment of his professorial functions, and the constantly recurring labor of revising either the Pharmacopoeia or the Dispensatory,—he had no inducement to new attempts at authorship, or in any other direction to seek for new fields of industry.

As a member of the Wistar Party, and the Senior Medical Club, he performed duly his function whether of host or of guest; participated in our anniversary Philosophical Dinners, then more fashionable than now; in all respects acted duly the part becoming his social position; and gave to the various associations and institutions, benevolent, scientific, or professional, with which he was connected the proper share of time and attention. Thus fully occupied, without being overworked, with no serious drawback to his comfort, he was, perhaps, as happy as is consistent with this uncertain state; and the current of his life, though somewhat agitated in its earlier course, now flowed onward copiously, richly, and smoothly to its end.

Having sufficiently detailed the incidents of his career, it only remains that I should endeavor to portray his qualities as a man. His mental qualities, though not peculiar in their nature, were in some respects strikingly so in degree, so as on the whole to constitute an extraordinary character. With little of the imaginative or inventive faculty, he had an excellent reason and judgment, and at least an average power of observation. He therefore seldom sought or made discoveries, never formed theories, except as convenient categories for facts, and generally eschewed figures of speech and flights of fancy, whether in speaking or writing; but he was almost always clear in thought and correct in conclusion, remarkably sound in his opinions, and seldom wrong in his judgments either as to the character and probable actions of men, or as to what was expedient under any given circumstances.

In mental action, as in his bodily movements, he was remarkably slow and deliberate, but was, therefore, all the less liable to error; and when his conclusions were once attained, he was even more slow to change than he had been to form them.

Though generally serious in thought and manner, he was possessed, in no slight degree, both of the sense and faculty of humor, which often rendered him a delightful companion, but his pleasantries partook of the quietness of his general deportment, were never boisterous or offensive, and rarely, if ever out of place. There was a singularly marked line of division between his serious and lighter veins; and, unlike many wits who never hold back a ludicrous thought, however grave the occasion, he almost never mixed the two together.

I have not known an individual who better illustrated the adage, *sapientis est desipere in loco*; who better knew, or, perhaps, I should rather say, more accurately felt when it was proper to be sober, and when to be playful and gay. But it was more in his moral than in his intellectual character that his peculiarities lay. Dr. Bache was apparently, rather by nature than by education, eminently conscientious. To believe that anything was right was, with him, as a matter of course, to act accordingly. The idea of doing what he believed to be wrong would seem not to have occurred to him; and the attractive appeared to lose its character when dissociated from the right, and to be no longer even tempting.

He had, moreover, a natural love of truth, justice, and method, perhaps essentially the same mental quality, differing only in application, as all are resolvable into the simple love of order; truth being the due relation of things in regard to fact, justice in regard to compensation or reward, and method in regard to position; so that one who by nature is very fond of order, will be apt to be true and just as well as methodical, unless perverted by accidental counterinfluence.

At all events, our deceased friend had all these qualities in an eminent degree. I never knew him to tell or even hint an untruth, to do an unjust act, or knowingly cherish an unjust thought; and every one acquainted with him, ever so slightly, must have been struck with the remarkable method and precision which pervaded all that he said or did.

Another conspicuous moral trait was a placidity of temper that was proof against almost any provocation; not that he did not feel an injury or injustice done, whether to himself or others, and express himself accordingly; but the feeling provoked was rather that of regret than of anger, and the offence was readily forgiven when not attended with some moral obliquity.

Taking him altogether, I never knew a man with a better balanced mind, or one who more nearly approached to my notions of perfection in all that concerns the moral character. As a consequence of his various excellences, and certainly without any purposed action of his own, for with all his amiable qualities he was remarkably independent, he conciliated almost universal good will; and few men have been more generally esteemed, and, where well known, better beloved than he.

Dr. Bache's writings and public teaching were marked by his characteristic intellectual traits. Simplicity, clearness, truthfulness, accuracy and method were their chief qualities, in regard both to material and arrangement. Correct reasoning and sound judgment were also evinced whenever there was occasion for their exercise. His style was easy and remarkably correct, even to the punctuation, and his language pure, idiomatic English. His published writings are entirely exempt from any appearance of effort or attempt at display. The purely ornamental is eschewed entirely. Figures of speech, flights of fancy, and flowers of rhetoric, are unknown to them.

In the spring of 1864, just as he was about to enter upon the task of preparing a new edition of the United States Dispensatory, which he expected to be peculiarly laborious, he was seized with an illness that proved to be his last. After considerable suffering for two or three days, his pains left him almost entirely, and in a few days more he sank into a state of prostration and stupor, which terminated in a perfectly easy death, on the 19th of March, somewhat more than a week from the commencement of the disease. He was in his seventy-second year when he died.

EDITORS' NOTE

Not mentioned in the memoir by Dr. Wood is Franklin Bache's keen interest in acupuncture. In fact he is credited with introducing it to the U.S. from Europe by his 1825 translation from the French of Morand's "Memoir on Acupuncture." Most American physicians were cautious about adopting it since it had the stigma of quackery. This may also be the reason Dr. Wood did not include it in his memoir. Franklin Bache seems to have been the most active proponent of the method. While he was a physician at the State Penitentiary he evaluated the use of acupuncture as a treatment for chronic pain in 17 prisoners who were suffering from various ailments including back pain, rheumatism, neuralgia, opthalmia and headache. His 1926 report in the North American Medical Surgical Journal claimed that 7 of them were completely cured, 7 considerably relieved and 3 unchanged. Over the next several decades acupuncture was attempted by several other well-known American doctors including Robley Dunglison (APS 1832) and William Osler (APS 1885). But Bache's enthusiasm for it did not prevail and except for Chinese practitioners its use died out.

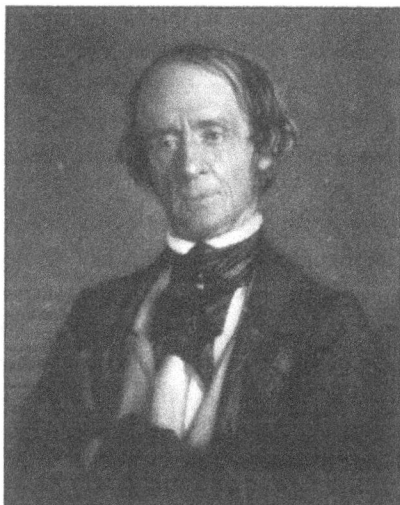

CHARLES D. MEIGS

1792–1869 (APS 1826)

Memoir by John Bell

Doctor Meigs was born February 19th, 1792, in the Island of Bermuda, where his parents had taken up their temporary abode, but in a few months after they returned to their native home in New Haven, Connecticut. At the age of seven years he accompanied his father to Athens, Georgia, on the occasion of the latter being made President of the College at that place. Under such favoring auspices the education of young Charles was carried on with the happiest results, as manifested by his knowledge of the Greek and Latin classics, in addition to that in other branches. He acquired, through an intimate intercourse with a French immigrant noble, a command of that language, so that he was able to speak and write it with great fluency and idiomatic accuracy.

During a portion of his boyhood his delicate frame and health gained strength and restoration by following the advice of his physician, that he should go for a season into the Cherokee country and participate to a certain extent in Indian life. Here he found in the person of one of the natives a companion and teacher in riding and shooting, whose extempore lessons were probably more effective for the purposes intended than formal instruction in the menage or cavalry drill. It was Chiron teaching the future follower of Esculapius.

He graduated at the University of Georgia in 1809. In the same year, 1809, Dr. Meigs began his medical studies under the instructions of Dr. Fendall (supposed in Augusta, Georgia,) to whom he was apprenticed for three years and took his degree of the Doctorate in the University of Pennsylvania, in the year 1815. His next step in life, to him in every way a fortunate one, was his marriage with Miss Mary Montgomery, of Philadelphia. From this union came a numerous issue, all of the members of which were estimable, some distinguished members of society.

The field chosen by Dr. Meigs for professional labor was Augusta, Georgia, and the selection was followed by every prospect of success, but the ill-health of Mrs. Meigs made him abandon his expectations and remove to Philadelphia. Through the temporary cloud of disappointment at his being obliged to change the theatre of action, even his sanguine nature would hardly prompt him at the moment to indulge in visions of professional fame and honors, which lay before him in a somewhat lengthened perspective.

He had, like most of those most distinguished in the annals of medicine, to undergo a period of probation, in which patients were the persons who in smallest number came under his notice. But, whilst waiting for business, he was neither an idle nor a querulous expectant, nor a lounger waiting for something to turn up, nor worse still, becoming a devotee of Bacchus and turning his back on the tutelary Apollo. In this early period of his life, Dr. Meigs took an active part in the discussions in the Philadelphia Medical Society, in participation with others of his compeers, who afterwards gained for themselves a name as writers and teachers. Among the early printed productions of his was the annual discourse before the Society, delivered February 18th, 1829.

He was one of the first to join in the formation of the Kappa Lambda Society, founded by Dr. Samuel Brown of Kentucky, in one of his annual visits, the only defect of which was its being for some time a secret one. Its objects were the elevation of the medical profession, increase of its usefulness, and the promotion of harmony and good fellowship amongst its members.

With this view it framed a code of ethics and brought out in 1835 a quarterly periodical called the North American Medical and Surgical Journal. It was the good fortune of the present writer as chairman of a committee on the projected Journal to be instrumental in having Dr. Meigs appointed one of its five editors; his associates in the work were, Drs. Bache, Coates, Hodge, La Roche, to whom were added at a subsequent period, Drs. Wood, Condie, and Bell.

To the pages of the North American Medical and Surgical Journal, which soon met with the favor of the profession, both at home and abroad, the subject of our memoir contributed his share in the shape of original articles, reviews and a portion of the Quarterly Summary. His department in this last was Midwifery,—an attribution which showed a great change in his own views and action respecting this important branch of Medicine.

In the first period of his career he carefully kept himself aloof from practising it, with an aversion scarcely less decided than that expressed by Lord Brougham against law, when it was a question whether to take it up as a profession, engage in the exclusive exercise or enter into public life. Writing from Edinburgh, Brougham says, that he still continues to detest his cursedest of all cursed professions; and some years later when in the Middle Temple, he tells Lord Gray, that there are few things so hateful as this profession; but nowithstanding this extreme repugnance, he became a member of the English Bar, went on the Northern Circuit, and concluded his legal career by being made Lord Chancellor.

Doctor Meigs was induced to change his course by the advice of judicious friends, who pointed out to him the advanced age of the prominent practitioners of Midwifery and the room that would ere long be left for younger aspirants. Accordingly he entered at once with his characteristic ardor the untried road, and soon began to win reputation for his assiduous attention and the skillful management of his patients,who were warm in their praises of their new accoucheur.

With a knowledge of his great sensibility and imaginative turn of mind, one can readily understand the effort it must have cost him to subject himself to the trials of patience, under the wearisome details, the anxiety and responsiblity which he continually encountered, in a still greater degree than in the ordinary practice of medicine, which of itself has a heavy load of cares to carry.

The explanation must be found in the very qualities of the man, which made him regardless of difficulties and obstructions in the excited determination to overcome them, in the lofty belief that he had become a ministering spirit endowed with the almost apostolic powers for the relief of those who placed themselves under his care, and appealed to him in their trouble. Once engaged in his mission, he gave himself no pause nor halted on the way, but steadily, cheerfully and kindly, at all hours and seasons, placed himself at the command of those who sought his services. If these were not always remembered with gratitude he did not complain, but consoled himself with the overflowing thankfulness and warm regard of those, and the number was continually increasing, who had been soothed and relieved by his ministrations.

Once fully engaged in the practice of Obstetrics he determined to make himself master of its literature, and with this view he set himself to a translation of Velpeau's Treatise on Midwifery, and projected an elementary work of his own on the same subject.

At an earlier date, and while still an editor of the Medical Journal, he had brought out a translation of Hufeland on Scrofula, in 1829, and in the same year as the annual discourse before the Philadelphia Medical Society. As we find him at this time, so he continued in the whole of his subsequent professional career, snatching at every interval left in his attendance on his patients to continue his studious life. Often would he, returning to his home from a detention through the greater part of the night in a sick-room, sit down to his desk and cheat himself of the few remaining hours till morning, in place of gladly taking the needed repose. This strain on mind and body carried with it the risk of a break down of both, and ambition's honors being lost when they are almost within grasp. Dr. Meigs in his reasoning process paid a heavy penalty for a neglect of the laws of nature in much severe suffering from an abdominal neuralgia, and also from a bronchial attack; but he rallied, regained his elastic bearing and customary strength, and resumed his onward course radiant and rejoicing to carry his sunshine of reviving spirit and skill into a long succession of sick-rooms.

On the breaking out of the Asiatic epidemic cholera in Philadelphia, in the summer of 1832, there was a call for the services of a number of her physicians to help to stay the pestilence and mitigate its violence. On such occasions medical men are always eager volunteers to encounter the assaulting fiend, in disregard of their ease and health, and ready to make the forlorn hope, and sacrifice their lives for the public good and safety.

No blast of trumpet, no beat of drum heralded the advance of the physician to the conflict; and no honors are awarded to his success, no commemorative monument raised to his memory if he falls a sacrifice to his duty. Within the short period of six months during which the yellow fever of 1793 raged with the greatest violence in Philadelphia, no less than ten physicians were carried off by the disease and scarcely one of the surviving members of the faculty escaped an attack.

In the famine year of 1847, in Ireland, one hundred and seventy-eight Irish practitioners, exclusive of medical students and army surgeons, died of the prevailing typhus fever, being a proportion of nearly seven per cent of the entire medical professional force of the country. The popular belief is that physicians have a kind of charmed life which gives them an immunity from the common causes of disease, and it is a matter of wonder that they bear up so well as they do under the various circumstances in which they are so continually placed.

Dr. Meigs was chosen to take charge of one of several temporary hospitals opened and fitted up by the city for the reception and treatment of patients who had no home nor the means of procuring suitable diet and nursing. In acknowledgment of their services, which happily were of short duration and unattended by mortality in their number, he, in common with each of his associates, received from the City Councils a silver pitcher.

A vacancy in the chair of Midwifery in the University of Pennsylvania was created by the broken health and subsequent resignation of Dr. Dewees; and Dr. Meigs presented himself as a candidate for the succession. The contest between him and his successful rival, Dr. Hugh L. Hodge, was animated and served to extend a knowledge of his professional and personal merits. His disappointment on the occasion was keen, but was soon compensated for by his receiving with, we believe, entire unanimity on the part of the Trustees of the Institution, the Professorship of Midwifery in the Jefferson Medical College in 1841. Three other chairs, viz.: of the Practice of Medicine, Chemistry, and Surgery, were filled at the same time by the election of Drs. John K. Mitchell, Franklin Bache, and Thomas D. Mutter; the other Professors were Drs. Joseph Pancoast, Robert M. Huston, and Robley Dunglison.

Under this re-organization of the Faculty, the fortunes of the Jefferson College, which in former years had been often clouded and adverse, became at once propitious and successful, and to this happy result it must be said with a full appreciation of the ability and attainments of his associates in the College, Dr. Meigs largely contributed.

His love for the beautiful was ingrained in his philosophy, and gave a coloring both to his written and spoken compositions, and the strongest instance of which is exhibited in his work, "Woman: Her Diseases and Remedies," in the form of letters addressed to his Class in 1848. The author describing to his readers her diseases and the means of cure presents a picture of woman with all her attributes, as a sentient, excitable and imaginative being, easily affected by the surrounding influences of sky and air and social habits, craving for admiration, affection and friendship, charming even in her smaller vanities, and noble in the devoted discharge of domestic and religious duties at every sacrifice. From her come the quickening spirit of the charities and amenities of the world, all that adds grace to civilization, and impels and sustains man in deeds of patriotism and practical philanthropy.

The author illustrates his view of woman's nature by drawing on physiology, psychology, classic love, and the collateral aids of poetry and the fine arts, with such happy adaptation as to make that which might at first seem to be diffuse and extraneous matter, appear to be a part of the general argument, not merely to show what woman is, but in what variety of channels the physician must carry his scrutiny, and what a variety of means he must enlist for the treatment of her maladies, compounded, as they so often are, of both bodily and mental troubles.

In his intentness to diffuse a knowledge of the subject as taught from his chair in Midwifery and the diseases of Women and Children, in the Jefferson Medical College, he spared no labor, and seemed to invite, as it were, literary and professional rivalry. His next original performance was a treatise entitled Obstetrics the Science and the Art, in 1849, which he wrought ex cathedra, with the weight of large experience and discriminative ability. Nearly simultaneous with the appearance of this volume was that on Child-bed Fevers. In the same year, which was that of the second visitation of epidemic cholera in Philadelphia, he gave in a brochure his thoughts on this disease, termed by him spasmodic cholera, for private distribution.

Next in order of time comes his volume on the Nature, Signs, and Treatment of Child-bed Fevers, in 1854. He strenuously advocated the non-contagiousness of Puerperal Fever, and the preference to be given to venesection in its treatment, in both of which views he subjected himself to much opposing inculcation, and severe, abusive criticism. He had, several years previously, indicated his creed on the subject, by introducing to the profession, by an introduction and notes, short monographs by Hay,

Armstrong, and Lee, in 1842. The Treatise on Child-bed Fevers was pronounced by the Edinburgh Journal to be superior to any one work upon the same subject.

Dr. Meigs was no silent member of the different societies with which he became connected. The Records of the Philadelphia College of Physicians, of which he was some years Secretary, the American Philosophical Society, and the Academy of Natural Science, bear proofs of his professional and scientific zeal. Notice has already been taken of the large share he had in editing and contributing to Chapman's Journal of Medical and Physical Sciences, and its successor in due sequence; the American Journal of Medical Science; also the Medical Examiner, and the New Orleans Medical and Surgical Journal.

Dr. Meigs, when Secretary of the College of Physicians of Philadelphia, introduced to that body two gentlemen from New England, delegates to represent in different quarters the flood of evil resulting from the use of intoxicating liquors, and to take measures for diminishing its violence and destructive effects, by discontinuing the use of distilled spirits. His own habits always temperate, and finding in a fervid imagination incentives to thought, he never sought the unnatural excitement of the bottle, and hence readily adopted the first steps in the temperance reformation, by his abstaining steadily from the use of distilled spirits and withholding them, as far as possible, from his patients. He did not carry his detestation of alcohol so far, however, as to inhibit its use in fermented liquors, and tobacco found in him a regular customer.

Dr. Meigs allowed himself but little respite from professional toil, and, with few exceptions, took no vacations, such as are of right, and almost of necessity, the practice of most medical men in the summer months. In the year 1842 he visited Mackinaw and the Falls of St. Anthony, to recruit his almost exhausted energies and in 1845 he visited Europe for a similar purpose. During a few months absence on this occasion, he made the acquaintance of many of the medical notabilities of France and England, who were prepared, by the reputation which he had acquired, and a knowledge of his works, to receive him with appreciative cordiality. In Paris he read a paper on Cyanosis, in French, before the Academy of Medicine, and received warm commendation from some of the members, not only for his very ingenious view of the subject, but for his good idiomatic and well-spoken language on the occasion.

At a later period, in his Treatise on Certain Diseases of Young Children, he enters into anatomical and physiological details, explanatory of the cause of Cyanosis, and of his new method of treating it. The novel feature in the latter consisted in turning the child on its right side, and slightly raising its head and shoulders. Several instances are given by the author of the success of this procedure, which, considering that Cyanosis occurs under different anatomical conditions of the heart, can only be expected to be serviceable in some of them.

In common with the majority of his fellow-practitioners in Philadelphia, Dr. Meigs was slow in having recourse to etherization in his Obstetric cases, and to the use of chloroform he was opposed to the last; and certainly not without reason, when scarcely a week passes but we hear of death from chloroform, when used as an anesthetic for women in tedious and painful labor, and for surgical operations, some of them of a very slight nature. And the question of anesthetics was discussed in letters between Sir James Simpson, of Edinburgh, and Dr. Meigs, a pleasant feature of which consisted in the courteous manner in which the parties treated each other.

The subject of this memoir had long sighed for freedom from his arduous duties of teacher and practitioner, and for leisure to indulge his literary tastes and his fondness for natural science. In proof of the sincerity of his intention to procure these enjoyments, he made preparation by purchase of a piece of land and the erection of a house, five miles beyond Media, in a beautiful region of country. He yielded with pleasant equanimity to the conviction that he was getting old, and determined to avail himself of the compensation which age brings with it.

The first step was diminishing his professional labor; the next, the resignation of his Chair in the College. This event took place after the course of 1859–1860, to the regret of his associates and the crowds of students all over the land, who had anticipated the pleasure and instructions from his predilections, on which those in advance of them had descanted so lovingly. At last Dr. Meigs found himself in the country-home of his own creation, and free to pass his time in the pleasures of his books and his garden. But a sad break was to be made in this united enjoyment by the death of Mrs. Meigs, which took place on May 13th, 1865.

Thus, in the midst of his loving family, the endearments of his friends, and the respect of the community, Dr. Meigs filled up the measure of his allotted days. His decease took place on the 22nd June, 1869, at the age of 77 years.

EDITORS' NOTE

As noted in the memoir Dr Meigs' treatise on child bed fever (1854) was well known and praised. This was unfortunate since his emphasis of the "non infectious" nature of the disease was influential. Not mentioned is the polemic Dr. Meigs carried out with a "scribbler" (Oliver Wendell Holmes, APS 1880). Meigs ridiculed him for proposing in his 1843 publication that hand washing by their obstetricians would save the lives of many women by preventing puerperal sepsis. Dr Meigs believed that doctors are gentlemen and a gentleman's hands are clean.

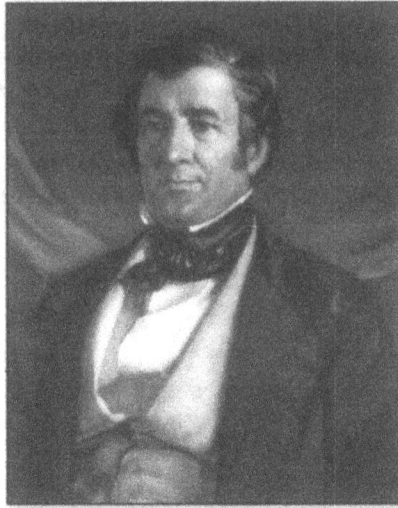

JOHN KEARSLEY MITCHELL

1793–1858 (APS 1827)

Memoir by Robley Dunglison

Dr. John Kearsley Mitchell was born in Shepherdstown, Virginia, on the 12th of May, 1793. His father was Dr. Alexander Mitchell, a native of Scotland, and a member of a respectable family in Ayrshire, who came to this country in 1789, took up his residence in Jefferson County, Virginia, and soon afterwards married into the Kearsley family, who resided at that time in Pennsylvania. Dr. Mitchell's father died before he was nine years old; and he was left in the charge of a guardian, who sent him to Scotland in 1807, to be educated. In the town of Ayr he received his early instruction, and it was here, in the land of Burns, that he imbibed that love for the simple, but eminently expressive productions of Scotia's bard, which led him, on many occasions, whilst, as he remarked, "he sat in his office and waited for practice," to indulge in poetical compositions, several of which were received with no little favour.

From Ayr he went to the University of Edinburgh, to complete his scholastic education, and in the year 1816 returned to America, and commenced the study of his profession with Dr. Kramer, of Jefferson County, Virginia, for whom he ever felt the greatest respect and veneration, and of whose character he often spoke enthusiastically in his lectures before the class of Jefferson Medical College. Subsequently, he became a pupil of Professor Chapman, of Philadelphia.

His studies were, however, interrupted by impaired health, which induced him to take a voyage to China, from which he returned much improved; and after having obtained his diploma in the University of Pennsylvania, in 1819, he twice repeated the voyage in the capacity of surgeon to a merchant vessel. On his return to America, he established himself in Philadelphia, and, early in 1822, married a daughter of Alexander Henry, Esq. In the same year he was appointed physician to the Almshouse Hospital, and, some years afterwards, to the Pennsylvania Hospital.

Between the years 1833 and 1838, he delivered a course of lectures on chemistry applied to the arts, in the Franklin Institute, and as early as the year 1822, formed part—as lecturer on medical chemistry—of the first summer association for teaching medicine, established in Philadelphia. He lectured, also, on physiology and on chemistry, for some years to a private class. In the year 1841, on the reorganization of the Faculty of Jefferson Medical College, he was looked to as eminently qualified to occupy the Chair of Practice of Medicine, to which he was accordingly appointed, and from that time forward ably fulfilled the various duties which appertained to it.

In the spring of 1856, he was attacked with hemiplegia, from which he gradually, but never wholly recovered. It did not, however, interfere with the active exercise of his professorial duties in the following winter. In the course of the subsequent session, he experienced a second but slighter attack, which did not prevent him from meeting his class for more than a week, and neither of them seemed to have impaired his intellect. He never, indeed, rendered the various services that devolved upon him as professor, with greater satisfaction to his hearers. In the latter end of March, 1858, he was attacked with typhoid pneumonia, which speedily terminated his existence, in the 65th year of his age.

In the various relations of life, Dr. Mitchell was highly and justly estimated. In his profession he was held in great regard. Kind and attentive to his numerous patients, he was looked upon as a valued friend, as well as cherished medical adviser; as a teacher of medicine, he was faithful and energetic, alive to every improvement, and ever anxious to imbue his pupils with the great principles of their profession, and with the divine art of applying these principles to practice; as a cultivator of general science, he was full of zeal; and whilst he was a lecturer on chemistry—and there are many who retain a vivid recollection of his merits as such—he was watchful for every suggestion of value, and hastened to adopt them, with modifications indicated by his own ingenious and fertile mind.

An example of this was the apparatus framed by him for the formation of solid carbonic acid. His researches, too, into the phenomena of capillarity, as exhibited in the penetrativeness of different liquids and gases, and the penetrability of different septa, and respecting which a philosopher of great distinction, Milne Edwards, of Paris, has very recently expressed his astonishment that they should have been treated with neglect by the greater part of physicists, were replete with interesting applications to physiology more especially.

As an author, he confined himself chiefly to Monographs, several of which were published in the scientific journals, and in detached pamphlets. To one on the penetration of gases, allusion has already been made. Others were on the formation of Solid Carbonic Acid Gas; on Air, Fire and Water, as illustrating the Wisdom and Goodness of God; a New Theory and Treatment of Rheumatism; on Curvatures of the Spine; on the Tests for the Detection of Arsenic; on the Smallpox; on the Means of Elevating the Character of the Working Classes; on the Value of the Practical Interrogation of Nature; on the Value of a Great Medical Reputation, &c. &c.

Several of these were originally delivered before the Franklin Institute or the Jefferson Medical College. He read, also, before the College of Physicians of Philadelphia, an interesting communication on the phenomena of mesmerism as observed by him, with the inferences which he drew therefrom.

His most elaborate monograph, however, was on the cryptogamous origin of malarial fever, which was replete with interesting facts and ingenious deductions. He published, also, an article in the American Cyclopedia of Medicine and Surgery, on the Chemical and Pharmaceutical History and Toxicological Effects of Arsenic, and edited the American reprint of Faraday's Chemical Manipulations.

Dr. Mitchell was the author of various other scientific and literary productions, which added to his well earned and well merited reputation; and was a member of many scientific, literary, and philanthropic institutions. He was elected into this Society in the year 1827.

EDITORS' NOTE

It is understandable that Robley Dunglison's 1858 memoir of John Kearsley Mitchell does not mention his son who at the time was only 29 and not yet famous. But only four years later his son, S. Weir Mitchell, had become famous as one of the U.S.'s most distinguished physiologists. He had also become a member of the APS.

In addition to 33 papers on various aspects of the circulation, respiration, muscle and reflex activity, S. Weir Mitchell with U.S. Surgeon General William Hammond (APS 1859) described the effects of venoms and toxins. During the Civil War with his junior colleagues John Morehouse (APS 1877) and WW Keen (APS 1884) he conducted and reported landmark studies on gunshot wounds and other injuries of nerves discovering he phenomena of causalgia and phantom limb syndrome. Later S. Weir Mitchell developed his famous "rest treatment" for psychiatric disorders. In addition to his extensive bibliography and international reputation on neurological and other medical disorders the younger Mitchell became even better known as one of the country's most widely read authors of fiction, publishing 15 novels and many other works, most dealing with historical or psychiatric themes. At the time of his death at age 84 he was Philadelphia's and perhaps the Nation's most honored physician and one of its best known citizens. S. Weir Mitchell is not included in this collection because no APS memoir of him was written.

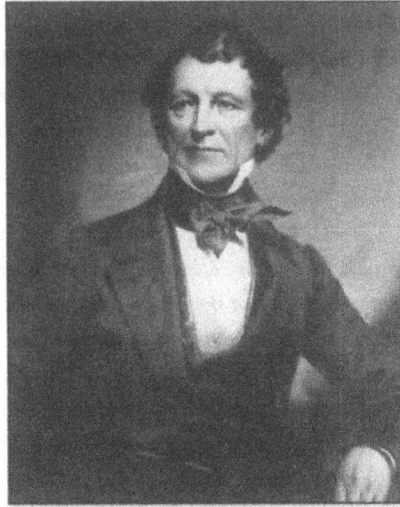

GEORGE B. WOOD

1797–1860 (APS 1829)

Memoir by Henry Hartshorne

He was born at Greenwich, in New Jersey, in the year 1797. His own memoranda of his ancestry are not devoid of historical interest in connection with the early settlement of this city, as well as that of our neighboring State. It appears that Richard Wood, a member of the Society of Friends, came to this country with William Penn in 1682, bringing with him his son James, and settled in the northern part of the then new city of Philadelphia; where Wood street probably received its name from him.

George B. Wood was the eldest son of Richard and Elizabeth Bacon Wood. At twelve years of age, his earnest desire for a liberal education was gratified by his father sending him to school in New York. When sufficiently prepared, he was transferred to the University of Pennsylvania, where he was graduated, with honors, in 1815.

Upon leaving the Collegiate Department of the University, young Wood began the study of Medicine as the office student of Dr. Joseph Parrish. His advantages there were decidedly superior; and he availed himself of them so well as to become, after his graduation in Medicine at the University in 1818, his preceptor's associate in giving instruction to students. A private medical school grew out of this association; in which a number of our most eminent physicians and surgeons, of the generation now passing away, took part, first as pupils, and some of them afterwards as instructors.

Under such circumstances, Dr. Wood matured those convictions upon practical medicine and medical ethics which he inculcated through his whole life; and which during the forty-two years of his continuous labors as a medical professor and clinical teacher, were spread broadcast throughout this country.

No one man has ever done so much as he, to form and influence medical opinion in America upon both practical and ethical questions. Well has it been for the profession, that his teaching was dictated by good judgment, careful study, and, above all, the highest principles of rectitude and honor.

Dr. Wood's first course of lectures was one upon chemistry, delivered to a non-professional audience, chiefly composed of ladies, in Dr. Joseph Parrish's private office. Here, in a lay course, as Dr. Littell observes, in a Memoir [Read before the College of Physicians of Philadelphia, October 1, 1879] to which I am much indebted for information, "before a class entranced by his carefully prepared experiments and not likely to be hypercritical in its judgments, he gained confidence and dexterity, and was thereby better fitted to perform his part in a more formal and important sphere." Shortly after the Philadelphia College of Pharmacy was founded, in 1821, Dr. Wood was invited to become its Professor of Chemistry. He accepted the position, and held it, with success and popularity, from 1822 to 1831, when he was transferred to the Chair of Materia Medica in the same institution.

In 1835, when the Chair of Materia Medica in the University of Pennsylvania (before held by Dr. John Redman Coxe) became vacant, Dr. Wood was elected to occupy it. I have had before me a letter addressed by him, during the canvass, to James S. Smith, one of the Trustees of the University, at the request of the latter, in which, with modesty and yet with distinctness, he sets forth some of the reasons, growing out of his abundant preparation, for his claim to the chair.

He mentions in this letter the fact, that during the year 1829 he devoted all his leisure for nine months, in conjunction with Drs. Hewson and Bache, acting as a committee of the College of Physicians, to the revisal of the Pharmacopoeia of the United States. So many alterations were found to be required, that it was necessary to rewrite almost the whole work. Before the Committee was satisfied, Dr. Wood states that he had written all of the manuscript copy at least twice over with his own hand.

Through its subsequent adoption by a National Convention at Washington in 1830, this Pharmacopoeia became the standard authority for the preparation of officinal medicines throughout the United States; and it has so continued, with repeated revisals, down to the present time.

Not long after completing this important work, Professor Wood began, with Professor Franklin Bache, aided for a time by Daniel B. Smith, then President of the Philadelphia College of Pharmacy, a very elaborate commentary upon the Pharmacopoeia, under the name of the United States Dispensatory. This, which made a volume of more than a thousand large and closely printed pages, was begun and finished by its authors in less than two years. It has, since that time, passed through fourteen large editions; the aggregate number of copies sold, during Dr. Wood's life-time, amounting to 120,000 copies; as it has long been regarded as everywhere indispensable to both the medical and the pharmaceutical professions.

The intimate association of Doctors Wood and Bache, in the preparation of this most useful work of reference, was only a part of the fabric of their life-long fraternal friendship. This close intimacy was the more remarkable on account of their being opposed in interest as professors in the two great rival medical schools; that of the Medical Department of the University of Pennsylvania, and the Jefferson Medical College of Philadelphia,

In the professorship of Materia Medica and Therapeutics in the University of Pennsylvania, Dr. Wood reached the culmination of his reputation as a public teacher. He was one of the leaders in that great reform in instruction upon scientific subjects, which has now become universal; in which illustration and demonstration, by the constant presentation of objects to the sight, are prominent and essential.

His courses of lectures upon Materia Medica may be truly said to have been splendid, almost magnificent; adorned as well as made complete for the students' information, by the exhibition, from day to day, of living specimens of medicinal plants from all quarters of the world, grown in his own private conservatory and botanical garden, maintained for this special purpose. When such could not at the time be obtained, fine pictorial representations were placed before the class in their stead; and his cabinet of mineral and other crude and prepared specimens was correspondingly complete.

A printed syllabus of the course of lectures, interleaved for note-taking, was furnished gratuitously by him to each student. It may be said, indeed, that no portion of the curriculum of the Medical Department of the University, able and renowned as have been the other members or its Faculty, ever added more to the great reputation and large classes of that institution, than this model course.

Dr. Wood continued to hold the Chair of Materia Medica and Therapeutics until 1850, when he was transferred to that of the Theory and Practice of Medicine, upon the retirement from the latter of Professor Nathaniel Chapman. This chair he retained until 1860, when he withdrew from all active professional labors.

Among other literary contributions of the earlier portion of Dr. Wood's professional life, one not without importance was, his taking prominent part in the editorship of the North American Medical and Surgical Journal. In 1835, Professor Wood was appointed one of the attending physicians to the Pennsylvania Hospital. The duties of this responsible post he performed, with unremitting faithfulness, until the year 1859. His clinical lectures in that institution, to numerous classes of medical students, were admirable.

Great improvements in the methods of ascertaining conditions of internal disease, and especially in the physical diagnosis of affections of the lungs and heart, were brought hither from Europe after Dr. Wood had begun his career as a medical teacher. Having no ultraconservatism in regard to novelties, he applied himself to the practical study of auscultation and percussion; so as to become proficient in their bedside use.

Not content, however, with his own skill in these newer methods, he availed himself, not unfrequently, of the assistance of the late Dr. W. W. Gerhard, with whom they were a specialty, in the diagnosis of cases under his care in the Hospital. It was one of Dr. Wood's characteristics, that, in his earnest and conscientious solicitude for the interests of his patients and pupils, he was always ready to supplement and extend the advantages of his own personal instruction, by engaging, upon the most liberal terms, the services of others in particular departments. This was constantly done by him in regard to his own private students, of whom, until about the year 1855, he always had a large class. Several of our most distinguished physicians, now leading practitioners and professors, can look back with grateful reminiscences to the hours advantageously spent, in review of their University studies, as Professor Wood's office pupils.

No event in Dr. Wood's life was of more cardinal importance to him than his marriage; which took place in 1823, to Caroline, only daughter of Peter Hahn, a wealthy merchant of Philadelphia. Congenial, domestic in her tastes, and devoted in her attachment to him, she was able, also, by her receipt of large means from her father, to secure her husband in an independent position in the world.

Some men would have availed themselves of this, to withdraw from care and toil of every kind, and to enjoy their leisure in travel and in social or literary recreation. Not so with Dr. Wood; while generous, and sometimes even stately, in his mode of living, he employed the resources placed within his reach mainly in enlarging and improving his processes of instruction; into which, as well as into the composition of his books, he threw all the energy of his nature.

Although without offspring, the companionship of his excellent wife was to him a constant source of happiness, until her death in 1865. With this loss, following that of Dr. Bache in 1864, began the decline of Dr. Wood's vigor, which slowly, and almost insensibly, proceeded, until his decease in the Spring of 1879.

In 1847, before his transfer to the Professorship of Practice of Medicine in the University, he published his great treatise, in two volumes, on the Practice of Medicine. This was at once recognized, at home and abroad, as an authoritative work. It became a favorite text-book for students, not only in this country, but also in Great Britain. The time-honored University of Edinburgh was one of several foreign medical schools in which it was officially approved and adopted. It passed, during its author's life, through six editions.

This work was followed, in 1856, by another, also in two octavo volumes, a treatise upon Therapeutics and Pharmacology. Of this, three editions were issued; the last in 1868. In both of these works, Dr. Wood showed the most indefatigable industry and excellent judgment, in research, selection and arrangement, of all the knowledge obtainable upon his subjects. In neither is there manifested much originality of invention or discovery or suggestion.

Dr. Wood's mental outlook was, indeed, far from being narrow, or in any sense restricted to matters connected with his own profession. He was earnestly and actively interested, for several years, in the establishment of Girard College according to the designs of its endowment.

In presenting this appeal to the public, after nine years had elapsed without any application of Stephen Girard's legacy to the education of orphans, it was understood that its author represented, although informally, the wishes of the Trustees of the College.

Shortly afterwards, Dr. Wood, as chairman of a committee of the same Board of Trustees, prepared a formal communication to the Select and Common Councils of Philadelphia, urging immediate action to carry out the provisions of Girard's will, by legal enactments and appropriations. The result of this conflict, however, between the Councils and the Board, was the dissolution of the latter, of which Nicholas Biddle was then President; and, also, the termination of the official connection with the College of its first President, Alexander Dallas Bache.

An important contribution was made, also, by Dr. Wood, to the organization of Girard College, in the form of a report of a committee of which he was chairman, upon the clothing, diet, etc., of its orphan pupils. This report comprised a brief but clear and systematic statement of the principles essential to the healthy conduct of such an establishment; such as, if carried out, must have secured to it from the start, excellent sanitary conditions.

Among other subjects upon which Dr. Wood wrote well, as he did upon all topics which interested him at all, was that of the Temperance reform. He contributed to the United States Review, in January, 1834, an article about fifty pages in length, on the "Temperance Cause." His views, in this article, were advanced for that day, although confined to an exposition of the evils attending the use of ardent spirits as a drink, and of immoderate indulgence in the use of fermented beverages.

That, with longer reflection and experience, his mind did not greatly change upon this subject, was shown by a note appended by him to a reprint of the above mentioned article, in 1872. "Were our efforts confined," he there says, "to the exclusion of ardent spirit or distilled liquors from use, there might be some hope of success in the end; as a people among whom temperance could be established, with this limitation, could never, so long as the rule continued, become a nation of drunkards."

Dr. Wood, while very fond of hospitality, and making his house a favorite social centre, especially for the members of his own profession, was a marked instance of the benefits of that temperance which he so ably defended and enjoined.

Historical composition always had a great attraction for Dr. Wood. In the two volumes of his Memoirs, Lectures and Addresses, published, the one in 1859, and the other in 1872, we find the following papers expressly of that character: History of Materia Medica; History of Materia Medica in the United States; Sketch of the History of the Medical Department of the University of Pennsylvania; History of the Pennsylvania Hospital, delivered at the centennial celebration of its foundation, with a supplement to this, delivered at the laying, in 1856, of the corner-stone of the new Penna. Hospital for the Insane; and a History of Christianity in India.

The last named of these historical memoirs was part of a larger plan of a history of India, conceived by its author in early life, and abandoned on account of the demands made upon his time by his professional duties. The eleven chapters which were completed make more than a hundred pages of the volume of Memoirs, &c., published by him in 1872.

There is added, also, as a supplement, an Address on the British East India Empire, which was delivered by Professor Wood before the Athenian Institute of Philadelphia, January 23d, 1839. From the latter, we may take, as bearing upon a topic whose interest to the world at large is increasing every year, the following concluding reflections:

> "But," it is there written, "the fortunes of India and Great Britain are not to be forever united. The English themselves, even those who have labored most assiduously in the consolidation of the Indian Empire, look forward to an ultimate separation. They look forward to the time, when, through the agency of causes brought to bear upon the people of India by their present political relations, they will have become enlightened, refined, elevated in sentiment and conduct; when the adoption of a pure religion will have cleansed away the moral foulness which now corrupts every spring of action; when their long union under one common government will have given them a feeling of political identity, a spirit of nationality and patriotism, which may lead them to desire independence, for which their expanded intelligence and purer morality shall have fitted them. When thus ripe for self-government, may we not reasonably hope, that India will fall off spontaneously and peaceably from her long attachment, and, either as one or as several people, take her place in that brotherhood of nations, which, in America, in Africa, and in Australasia, will have owed their origin or civilization directly or indirectly to Great Britain, and will continue to revere the name and cherish the institutions of this mother of empires, when she herself shall have fallen into the decrepitude of age, or have gone to join her predecessors in the realms of history?"

Of scientific contributions by Dr. Wood to the Proceedings of the American Philosophical Society, I find record of four. The first of these was delivered as an address to the Society, in 1860, his second year of service as its President, upon "Dangers of Hasty Generalization in Science." It exemplified, as well as inculcated, that cautious, although never timid spirit, which becomes the true philosopher; which welcomes the appearance of every promising novelty, in science or in art, but always refuses to accept it simply because it is new; which believes everything which is proven by sufficient evidence, but nothing without evidence, whatever its attraction to the fancy, the intellect, or even the moral sense.

Dr. Wood's other papers, published in the Proceedings of this Society, were upon the subject of his observations and experiments, carried on through several years, upon his farm at Greenwich, in regard to the fertilizing and renewing action of the alkali potassa on the growth of fruit-trees, potatoes, wheat and other plants. The addition of wood ashes empirically to certain soils under cultivation, has long been a common practice in many places.

By the chemical analysis of plants and of the earth in which they grow, as Dr. Wood mentions, their mutual physiological relations have, especially since the investigations of Liebig, been generally understood. But the merit of Dr. Wood's observations is, that they have furnished means of definite experimental demonstration, upon a considerable scale, of the practical application of this part of the chemical physiology of plants, in a manner productive of direct agricultural and horticultural profit.

In 1848, he was elected President of the College of Physicians of Philadelphia; an office which remained with him thereafter until his death. In 1855, he was made President of the American Medical Association; and in 1859, President of the American Philosophical Society. In 1870, Dr. Wood was disposed to retire from all official duties, on account of his advancing age and infirmity. On the occasion of his tendering his resignation of the presidency of the American Philosophical Society, its Secretaries were authorized, as a committee, to request its withdrawal. In the communication addressed to him in regard to it by them, he was assured on behalf of the members of the Society, that all continued to recognize him as "the most worthy representative it could have, not only where it holds its meetings, but in its correspondence with other learned bodies like itself."

His distinctions were not confined to his own city. The College of New Jersey bestowed upon him the degree of LL.D. Besides being made honorary or corresponding member of the New York Academy of Medicine, and the Medical Societies of Massachusetts and Rhode Island, the same honor was conferred upon him by the Société de Pharmacie of Paris, the Medico-Chirurgical Society of Edinburgh, the Royal College of Physicians of Dublin; the Silesian Society for Native Culture of Breslau, L'Accademia dei' Quiriti of Rome, and the Societas Caesarea Naturae Curiosorum of Moscow, Russia.

He attended, as a guest, two meetings of the British Association for the Advancement of Science, in 1848 and 1861. In the former year, he was appointed delegate from the American Medical Association to the meeting, at Bath, of the British Medical Association. At his reception on this occasion, when his credentials were read, complimentary resolutions were passed, and the whole assembly rose to greet him, as the accredited and honored representative of his profession in America. During his last visit to England, in 1861, appropriate official and social courtesies were extended to him, as President of the American Philosophical Society, and of the College of Physicians of Philadelphia, by the officers and members of the Royal Society, and of the College of Surgeons and Physicians in London.

Three journeys to Europe were made by Dr. Wood, in 1848, 1853, and 1860-61-62. He visited in turn nearly all the principal countries of Europe, including Russia. Nor were these, to him, tours only of idle amusement or mere recreation. His natural and acquired industry, his real love of work as well as of knowledge, induced him to study carefully, sometimes almost exhaustively, every place and object of interest.

A scientific note book was also kept by him, upon some particular subjects of interest and importance. Full, often elaborately detailed accounts of his observations are given, of the most varied things and places; as, for example, the Museum of Northern Antiquities at Copenhagen, to the description of whose contents he gives fifteen letter-size pages of his Journal; the geological structure and indications of the banks of the Tiber; art galleries and the carnival in Rome; vineyards and vine culture near Perugia, on the way from Rome to Florence; the Lariboisiére Hospital at Paris; the great International

Exhibition at London; the reception of a deputation of philanthropists by Lord Palmerston; and the annual dinner of the British Medical Association. One of the pleasing minor incidents of his last visit to London, was the refusal of the proprietor of a leading drug establishment in that city to receive payment from him for some rather expensive medicines, on account of the services rendered to himself by Dr. Wood in his writings.

Another, and still nearer, cause of anxiety began, early in the same year, to throw, as he wrote in his Journal, a deep shadow over Dr. Wood's future. This was the discovery that a cancerous tumor was beginning to threaten his wife's health and life. His plans of travel were altered in consequence. A voyage to Athens, Constantinople and Egypt was given up; and after some farther stay in Italy, the party traveled slowly toward Paris.

There, after careful surgical consultation, in April, 1862, the operation of excision was skilfully performed by the veteran surgeon, Velpeau, assisted by Nelaton, and Dr. Beylard, then of Paris, but formerly of Philadelphia. Dr. Wood's feeling upon the subject of his wife's illness and suffering was expressed thus in his Journal: "She and my country are the objects nearest my heart; and, if I know myself, I would willingly give up my own life, could I thereby secure the continued enjoyment of life and happiness to either." Her life was prolonged, with tolerable health for a considerable period, until 1865.

Before Dr. Wood's embarkation upon his last journey abroad, in 1860, a farewell public dinner was given him by members of the medical profession in Philadelphia, in testimony of their high respect, esteem and affection. The venerable and distinguished Dr. La Roche presided. The occasion was one of unusual interest. No physician in Philadelphia was ever more, if ever one so much, looked up to by those of all ranks and ages, as truly the head, the patriarch of the medical profession in America.

In person, Dr. Wood was rather tall; until the last few years of his life slender, and very erect in carriage. His features were regular, though not striking; he wore a peruke, and no beard. He was always dressed in black, and very neatly. His manners were dignified and formal; his whole appearance grave and sedate. To strangers, and those of slight acquaintance, he seemed rather to repel approach, and to produce a feeling of constraint.

Among intimate friends, however, in social intercourse, this severity was relaxed; so that, although never demonstrative, he was quite affable, and, at times, genial. As Dr. Packard describes him, in his brief biographical sketch [Transactions of the American Medical Association, 1879], "whoever learned to know him found in him a faithful friend, a judicious counsellor, and a true man." His uniform courtesy entitled him to be designated, as he was at the dinner given to him by the profession in 1860, "the model gentleman."

His conversation was agreeable and often very instructive, though not brilliant. In one respect, he was extremely different from Dr. Nathaniel Chapman. Twice only, in very frequent professional and social intercourse, did I hear him utter a facetious remark; and, then, it was rather the dry wit which brings a smile than the humor which compels laughter.

Open-handed benevolence was a marked trait of Dr. Wood's character. Privately, and to public institutions, he gave largely, although always with careful discrimination and judgment. The University of Pennsylvania, the Pennsylvania Hospital, the Philadelphia College of Physicians, the American Philosophical Society and the Academy of Natural Sciences were the main recipients of his liberal donations during his lifetime; and several of these institutions also became principal legatees in his will.

In all things, correctness, exactitude, method, and thoroughness were leading aims with Dr. Wood. These were shown above all other traits in his courses of instruction, private and public. No pains were spared to make every lecture complete, even in its smallest minutiae. His manner as a lecturer was comparatively quiet, but sufficiently energetic; with enough animation always to secure attention, although never in the least approaching rhetorical excess. Others might easily obtain more admiration for their eloquence; no lecturer in the University was ever more effective, in conveying instruction and information to his classes. Especially in the abundance and excellence of the illustrations accompanying his lectures, he was in advance of almost all his contemporaries.

But we must hasten towards our conclusion. To Dr. Wood, better than to most men, might be applied the poet's line: Justum et tenacem propositi virum.

If he had genius, it was a genius for work; a rare capacity for continued, indomitable, all-conquering labor. With this, he became an eminently successful man.

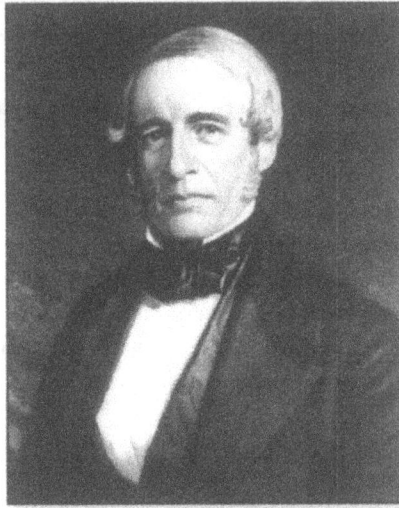

ISAAC HAYS

1796–1879 (APS 1830)

Memoir by Donald G. Brinton

The subject of the present memoir, Dr. Isaac Hays, had been at the time of his death, a member of this Society for very nearly fifty years, his name first appearing upon its rolls in 1830. For many years he was also one of the its most active members, and in the published volumes of our Proceedings which embrace the period previous to 1850, his name frequently recurs. Most of the subjects which he brought before the Society, related to medical science, and especially those portions of it connected with the physiology of visions and ophthalmic surgery.

But he did not confine himself to professional topics. I find, on looking over the earlier numbers of our Proceedings that he took considerable interest in geology, particularly in the remains of the gigantic mammals preserved from the post-tertiary period. About 1840, a number of such remains were collected in Missouri by Dr. Koch, and subsequently exhibited in this city and London. An active discussion arose among palaeontologists as to their classification. Besides the mastadon, the Elephas primagenius, and the mammoth, they distinctly proved, so one party maintained, the former existence of another species of mastodontoid animals belonging to the class Proboscidae, to which was given the name Tetracaulodon.

Dr. Hays sided with this party, and in addition to many verbal statements embodied in the Proceedings, he published in the Transactions a paper on the teeth of the mastodon, evincing in its preparation a most careful study of his theme. That later investigations have disproved his position, detracts but little from its merit; for the abstract correctness of a scientific theory is of less importance than the honesty and ability with which it is advocated. At various periods Dr. Hays served on the Committee of Publication, and the council, and was Curator.

At the time Dr. Hays was elected to this Society, he was thirty-four years of age. He was born July 5, 1796, in this city, his father residing at that time on Chestnut street below Third. His education had been first at the Grammar school kept in those days by Samuel Wylie, next at the University of Pennsylvania, whence he was graduated, A.M., in 1816; and finally as a medical student in the same institution whence he received the degree of M.D., in 1830. His preceptor was the eminent Dr. Nathaniel Chapman, celebrated not less for his wit than for his professional skill.

In early life Dr. Hays was much interested in natural science, and even before his graduation in medicine, he joined, in 1818, the Academy of Natural Sciences. With its history and success, he was identified for more than half a century. From 1865 to 1869 he was its President, and in many other official capacities actively aided its progress and influence.

His sympathies with the advance of general science led him to unite with others in the organization of the Franklin Institute. He was one of its original members, and for a number of years its Corresponding Secretary. To his activity much of the success of that prosperous institution can justly be ascribed.

As a physician, Dr. Hays studied and practiced his profession to a spirit of liberal culture and honorable feeling. The special branch which he cultivated was ophthalmology, and for a long time he stood first in that department in this city. He was one of the earliest to detect the pathological condition known as astigmatism, and the case which led to his discovery of it was reported to this Society.

His professional life was not confined to the care of his large practice, but extended to the relations of medical men to each other and to the public. Thus he was a member of the Convention which organized the American Medical Association, and of that which led to the formation of the State Medical Society of Pennsylvania. As Chairman of the committee of the former body to draw up a Code of Ethics, he was mainly instrumental in collating and reporting the code which has since been universally adopted throughout this country, and in some parts of Europe. He was also Chairman of the Board of Publication, and Treasurer of the Association for several years.

In September, 1835, he was elected a member of the College of Physicians and for a number of years was its Senior Censor. He was also Chairman of its Building Committee, and it was largely through his endeavors that the commodious structure at the corner of Thirteenth and Locust street, was erected for the College. Dr. Hays' literary labors include an edition of Wilson's Ornithology, 1828; Arnott's Elements of Physics, 1848; and some other medical works; but he is best known in this connection as the editor of the American Journal of the Medical Sciences, with which he was actively connected from February 1827, until his death. The ability and judgment he displayed in this task met with full recognition from the profession, both in this country and Europe, and the Journal has for half a century been recognized the world over as unsurpassed by any other medical periodical of its class in this country.

Advancing age led to his retirement from active practice in 1864-5, but he continued his literary and scientific labors, with unimpaired faculties and undiminished interest in the progress of knowledge to the last.

In conclusion, I may add that Dr. Hays married in 1833, and at his death left four children, one of whom is a prominent member of the same profession, and has succeeded to his father's position as editor of the American Journal of the Medical Sciences.

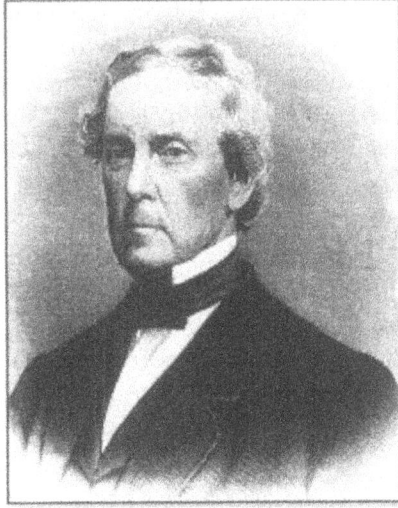

GOUVERNEUR EMERSON

1796–1874 (APS 1833)

Memoir by William Samuel Warthman Ruschenberger

At an early age he was sent to the Westtown School, a famous boarding school under the direction of the Society of Friends, which was opened May, 1799, in Westtown township, Chester county, PA. He returned to Dover, Kent county, Del. in 1810, and was for a short time at a boarding school in Smyrna, Del. Thence he was transferred to a classical school at Dover, the principal of which was the Rev. Stephen Sykes.

With the preliminary education acquired at those schools, and prompted by his mother, he began to study medicine at the age of sixteen, 1811, under the preceptorship of Dr. James Sykes, a prominent surgeon and eminent citizen, who was a first cousin of his mother. Dr. Sykes was once Governor of the State of Delaware, and during many years presided in its Senate. His father, Jonathan Emerson, died in 1812, leaving his family an ample real estate, consisting of farms and improvements thereon.

Gouverneur continued his study and went to Philadelphia, probably in the autumn of 1813, to attend medical lectures. Having attended three complete courses of lectures and submitted an inaugural thesis on Hereditary Diseases, the University of Pennsylvania granted Gouverneur Emerson, March, 1816, the degree of Doctor of Medicine. He was a member of the Philadelphia Medical Society from 1813, and was elected its Secretary in 1816.

Prior to his graduation he was a private pupil of Dr. Thomas Chalkley James, an eminent practitioner, who was professor of midwifery, the first ever appointed, in the University. During this association a warm and enduring regard sprang up between them. Dr. Robert Hutchinson Rose had purchased, in 1809, a hundred thousand acres of wild land, which included the township of Silver Lake, near Montrose, the capital of Susquehanna county, Pa., and was endeavoring to attract settlers upon it. He and Prof. James were cordial friends. Possibly influenced by the Professor's good opinion of his young friend, Dr. Rose invited Dr. Emerson to be his family physician, to become a member of his household, and practise medicine in the neighborhood.

Dr. Emerson arrived at Silver Lake about the end of September or beginning of October, 1816. He was a tall, slender man just past the twenty-first anniversary of his birth, and was, no doubt, hopefully forecasting the future of his career. Before he received Dr. Rose's invitation he had designed an excursion to the Northern States. After a survey of the position he was to occupy, he determined to delay beginning his work until after he had made his projected journey. He started alone on horseback from Silver Lake, October 15, 1816, and at the close of the next day reached Unadilla, a New York village, not very many miles beyond the northern boundary of Pennsylvania. He visited Schoharie, Schenectady, the Balstown Spa, Saratoga, and, passing over the Hudson river at Fish Neck, entered Vermont. From Rutland he crossed the Green Mountains to Montpellier and Danville; passed several days in Southern Canada, traversed New Hampshire and the province of Maine, and returned by the way of Waterford, Troy and Albany, to Silver Lake, after a ride of about 2000 miles. Dr. Emerson, who was probably the first physician settled there, practised his profession at Silver Lake nearly two years.

At the instance of a friend, Mr. Andrew Hodge, he was appointed, November, 1818, surgeon of a merchant ship, called the Superior, Captain John Hamilton, bound to China. He joined the vessel, which had already dropped down the river, December 7, 1818. The weather was stormy and the wind adverse. The Superior did not get to sea till the 12th. On the 13th, out of sight of land, a brig from Prince's Island, coast of Africa, bound to Rhode Island, was spoken. She had been seventy days at sea and was short of water. As the quarantine laws were then very rigidly observed at Marseilles, the port to which the Superior was bound, to avoid risk of vitiating her clean bill of health which might be consequent upon direct personal communication with any vessel or place before reaching Marseilles, casks of water were thrown overboard and picked up by the brig. On the 14th, being then in the Gulf stream, the doctor notes in his journal the use of the thermometer in navigation.

January 26, 1819, the Superior arrived at Marseilles, thirty-five days from the Capes of the Delaware. As soon as the ship entered the mole, the captain went to the Health Office, but was required to remain in his boat outside of the grate, and to throw his papers into a tub of vinegar presented to him, the object being to destroy any contagious matter they might contain. Letters brought for persons on shore, after being cut through in several places to give easy access to the vinegar, were treated in the same manner. Every vessel arriving was required to undergo quarantine. No person was permitted to land, and none to visit her from the shore. A guard was stationed on board to enforce observance of the rules. At the time the plague prevailed in the Barbary States.

A celebrated Dutch physician, Boerhaave, recommended distilled vinegar as an efficient remedy against putrid diseases. Vinegar was supposed to be antiseptic and therefore protective against all contagions. The hands of those who had to do with contagion were moistened with it, and their clothing and other objects were exposed to its vapors. During the plague of 1720, at Marseilles, it is said that four convicted thieves, who were employed in caring for the sick, protected themselves from the contagion by the use of vinegar, and were granted their lives on condition that they would reveal the means they used to shield themselves in their perilous work. And hence, perhaps, came the preparation called "Thieves' vinegar." But since modern studies of the processes of fermentation and putrefaction have led to the belief that they, as well as all contagions, are due to the presence of microscopic organisms, vegetal or animal, called mycroderms, bacilli, microbes, etc., vinegar has lost its antiseptic reputation.

Early on the morning of February 4, the harbormaster came alongside of the Superior. Learning from the guard that no one on the ship was sick, he came on board; and, after disinfecting the officers and passengers in the cabin and the sailors in the forecastle, by exposing them to the pungent fumes of oxymuriatic acid gas (chlorine), he granted pratique, i.e., liberty of the port. Then the ship was moved to the vicinity of the Custom House, and the gentlemen found quarters at the Hotel des Ambassadeurs.

After a sojourn of two months at Marseilles the Superior sailed April 5, and on the 15th anchored in Gibraltar bay; and was detained some time in quarantine, and afterwards many days waiting for a favorable wind. Before daybreak, May 6, 1819, the anchor was weighed and on the 7th the ship was fairly at sea.

August 1, the ship was anchored at Angier, Java, and on the 3d proceeded on her way. The anchor was let go again, Aug. 20, off Macao, where merchant ships bound to Canton were detained twenty-four hours. In the afternoon of the 21st a passport to proceed up the river was granted and a pilot sent on board. The ship started about half-past three o'clock P.M., and anchored in the Bocca Tigris sometime after midnight. The pilot landed the next morning to exhibit at the fort there the "chop" or permit to go up the river, and brought back two pilots and two Mandarins to remain on board till the ship reached Whampoa, the common anchorage of foreign ships trading at Canton. It is sixteen miles below the city. The Superior anchored in the evening of the 23d, and on the 26th, Dr. Emerson and fellow-voyagers were lodged in Swedes Factory at Canton.

He relates that in consequence of drinking Samshoo, a liquor prepared from rice, which in excess produces a fierce, maniacal intoxication, the crew of the Superior mutinied, and, in the absence of the captain, endeavored to kill the officers and take possession of the ship. Officers of other vessels lying near, immediately joined in the conflict. Some of the crew were knocked down and others stabbed. Eight of the ringleaders were put in irons, and fed on bread and water for ten days; and under such treatment became as subordinate as they always had been.

He gives an account of an accident to himself which might have been serious, as follows: "I went on board a ship where they kept a Spanish bloodhound. He was tied before I went on deck; but while sitting in conversation with some of my friends, he broke loose and sneaking alongside leaped into my face. The damage I sustained was a wound through the left lower eyelid, a deep cut on the temple, and one under my shoulder, together with a very black and inflamed eye, from all of which, I am happy to inform you, I have recovered. The dog is the most savage of his species. I escaped very well considering. He has injured others more seriously."

Referring to mosquitoes, he says: "I sleep under a net which lets the air circulate, but keeps out every kind of insect You will be pleased to see it. I think the plan so ingenious and good that it will be adopted by many of our friends." A plain implication from the Doctor's remark is that the mosquito net was a novelty to him in 1819, and not known in the neighborhood of his native place. Are we indebted to the Chinese for this invention?

The party finally left Canton for Whampoa, Nov. 22. The ship had been moved below the common anchorage when they reached her about noon. She arrived at Lintin on the 23d, and there found the U. S. frigate Congress, Capt. John D. Henley, said to have been the first American man-of-war to visit China. She anchored here Nov. 3, with many of the crew suffering from dysentery, ascribed to the water taken on board at Angier. Her presence aroused the suspicion of the Chinese authorities that it meant no good, and therefore they would not allow provisions to be furnished to her from Canton. The Superior brought several barrels of bread for her use, and other American merchantmen conveyed to her barrels of beef and pork.

On the 26th Nov. the Superior sailed from Lintin homeward bound. On Saturday, Jan. 16, 1820, then in the Indian ocean, she was boarded from a Patriot privateer, said to be two months out from Buenos Ayres. She was armed with sixteen guns and had a crew of two hundred men. Dr. Emerson, in his journal, says: "We first discovered her on Friday morning, about three miles off our starboard quarter, standing on the same course. The wind was light and unfavorable; a high head-swell further impeded our progress. Towards night the strange sail had gained upon us. We thought she showed a desire to speak. Every precaution seemed to have been taken to disguise her real character, by carrying little sail, but we still suspected her of foul intentions. The night was dark, but she kept close to us and always in sight. In the morning, being off our weather quarter, within gunshot, she ran up a Spanish flag and fired a gun to bring us to. When close to us she backed her topsails, hauled down the Spanish and ran up the Patriot colors, at the same time opened all her weather ports, ran out her guns and brought her whole broadside of eight guns to bear upon us. The star-spangled banner floated over our quarterdeck.

"We now thought ourselves in a rather unpleasant situation. Although no declared enemy, still the many outrages and pirates under what was called the Patriot flag made us fear we might not fare better than others under similar circumstances. "Her boat, rowed by a set of cutthroat-looking fellows, came alongside. The officer, apparently of inferior rank, wore a belt full of pistols and daggers. He was without a coat and barefooted. A renegade American attended him as interpreter. Having noted the ship's name, the latitude and longitude, etc., this accomplished officer directed his attention to our breakfast table, at which we had just intended to sit down. After refreshing himself and companions, the work of plunder began. They robbed us of many barrels of beef, pork, bread, butter, tea, silk, canvas, iron kettles, live stock, etc. The villains seemed to think themselves as fairly entitled to what they took as if they were purchasers. Whenever they came across anything they fancied, they said with all effrontery imaginable, 'Half for us and half for you,' adding from time to time, by way of consolation, 'We don't want to do you any harm.'

"They stated that they had a great deal of sickness on their ship and were throwing men overboard every day. They tried to induce me to join them, offering any rate of wages I might ask. They had a surgeon, but he was so indifferent that if in my way they would throw him overboard, and so get rid of him. His pay was a hundred dollars a month, but they would allow me any price I asked. Having consulted among themselves aside, they said that they had agreed not to force me to go with them against my will, although they were so much in want of medical assistance. According to their account the prevailing diseases on board were scurvy, dysentery, fever and ague, which had reduced what remained of the crew to a deplorable condition. Receiving a decidedly negative answer from me to their invitation, they next demanded a supply of medicines. I gave them some of a common kind, such as I thought might be useful to the wretches. The suspicious rascally officer took some of each one on the point of a dagger and thrust it into my mouth, watching me intently all the while, not satisfied till he had seen it on my tongue. This experience reminded me of a ludicrous scene in the "Honeymoon," where the doctor is forced to take his own medicine or be thrown out of the window.

"Though they robbed us in this unwarrantable manner, we were not treated as badly as we had expected. A strong breeze sprang up which prevented their small boats from passing between the two vessels. They permitted us to make sail, but followed in our wake. The breeze stiffened to a gale. Night came, dark and stormy. We changed our course. On the following morning, to our great joy, nothing was seen of our piratical friend."

March 20, the Superior was boarded by a Delaware pilot, and in the evening of the 23d reached Chester, 117 days from Lintin. The ship had been absent from Philadelphia sixteen months. His journal during the voyage contains testimony of industrious study and intelligent observation of all things at sea or on shore that impressed their images on his mind. Marine animals and aquatic birds, wherever they appeared were described. Drawings of some were made. These and original sketches of places seen, and maps of ports visited, with now and then an apt quotation from some poet, illustrate his pages.

He gives detailed accounts of what he saw at Marseilles and on his way to it. Whatever was new to the young traveler seemed to be charming. Appearances of people and things, famous localities with their historical associations combine to quicken curiosity and impart a glow of interest to his record of pageants viewed, of visits to hospitals, public buildings, theatres, museums, etc. Days were passed at Aix, St. Remy, Nimes, Avignon and Vaucluse. Many pages are given to descriptions of the remains of ancient Roman buildings, and of whatever interested him in those places. He gives interesting accounts of Gibraltar, and describes a visit with a companion on horseback to Algeciras, a port of Andalusia, six miles west of the famous fortress.

At Angier, in the Straits of Sunda, he tells of the many canoes and boats which came to the ship with fowls, fruits in great variety, vegetables, Java doves and Java sparrows in little bamboo cages, monkeys, paroquets, sea shells, and animals of the deer kind not taller than our domestic cat, and all being at moderate prices found ready sale among strangers. The natural, corporal characteristics of the Malays, seen here, their costume, language, as well as the appearance of their dwellings on shore, the mountain scenery, tropic vegetation, and political condition are sketched and commented upon. Macao, Whampao, Canton, Lintin; pagodas, scenery and Chinese boat population along the river are in like manner noticed in detail. The instruction derived from his observation and study, and the formative influence of his experiences during those months of separation from home, may not be definitely measured, but possibly to his alert mind they were as effective as the training of a college course.

With such preparation for work, on the 4th of August, 1820, the twenty-fifth anniversary of his birth, Dr. Emerson settled himself at No. 37 Chestnut street, Philadelphia, ready to give professional attention to any who might ask it. Possibly the time might have been opportune to introduce a young physician to business. Thirteen deaths from yellow fever in the city had been reported during the season of 1819. The circumstance had created a vague apprehension of its recurrence, and may have induced people to appreciate practitioners of medicine more highly than when there was no prospect of needing them; and consequently, new candidates for practice might be more promptly noticed. The apprehension was realized to some extent; during the autumn of 1820, seventy-three persons died of the disease in the city.

Dr. Emerson was appointed an attending physician of the Philadelphia Dispensary, September 19, 1820, and resigned the office, May 21, 1822. The City's Councils elected him a member of the Board of Health, March 12, 1823; and the Board appointed him its Secretary the same day. It is conjectured that he resigned three years later. Prevention of the introduction and spread of smallpox in the city at that period attracted attention. Between January, 1818, and December, 1822, five years, only nine deaths from smallpox in the city had been reported. Fear that the disease might again enter the city was no longer manifest. For this reason it was supposed that vaccination had been generally neglected in the community. The Board of Health was without authority to enforce measures to prevent the spread of the disease, then present, and for this reason its members were not willing to act; but at the instigation of Dr. Emerson the Board announced in the daily newspapers, three times, that smallpox was in the city and recommended all unprotected persons to be vaccinated without delay.

The same year, November 15, 1823, the Board again warned the public of its danger, saying "And as it is believed that there does exist among some an unjust prejudice against the practice of vaccination, the Board conceives it a duty to declare that the evidence afforded by our city in its long exemption from smallpox, together with the happy results which have followed the introduction of vaccination in all parts of the world, ought to be sufficient to convince the most incredulous of the salutary influence of this inestimable preventive."

Dr. Emerson submitted to the Board for approval and transmission to the Legislature a draft of a law and memorial on the subject. The proposed law in substance provided that vessels having smallpox on board should be quarantined on arrival in the same manner as those affected with other contagious diseases; that inoculation of smallpox should not be practised in any case without the sanction of the Board; and that authority already conferred on the Board of Health to deal with contagious diseases specified should be extended to smallpox.

After debating the subject at several meetings, the Board approved the memorial and draft of the proposed law, January 28, 1824, and transmitted them to the Legislature then in session. Although 160 deaths from smallpox had occurred in the city during 1823, a member of the House of Representatives retarded its action on the bill after it had passed the Senate by securing a seemingly innocent amendment to it, but which in fact provided that appointment to offices connected with the Board of Health might be so made as to reward political and partisan services without regard to fitness of the candidate. Mr. William Binder and Dr. Emerson were sent to Harrisburg to point out the effect of the amendment, and at the end of four days' work they secured its rejection and the enactment of the original bill. A copy of the act was duly delivered to the Board of Health, April 7, 1824.

His work as a member of the Board of Health, and his communications to the newspapers pointing out the risk of permitting those affected with smallpox to freely mingle with citizens, bear witness to Dr. Emerson's disinterested benevolence. During 1824, deaths from smallpox in the city numbered 325. They were reduced to six in 1825, and to three in 1826. But these facts are not conclusive that the measures taken by the Board of Health during this period contributed to abate the prevalence of the disease, because, both prior and subsequent to this time, the rate of mortality from smallpox in the city, between 1807 and 1840, fluctuated in the same striking manner, as Dr. Emerson shows in his papers on Medical and Vital Statistics, published in "The American Journal of the Medical Sciences," November 1827, November, 1831, and July, 1848.

In July 6, 1832, Dr. Emerson, accompanied by Dr. Isaac Hays, visited the first case of "spasmodic cholera" that occurred in the city, his original description of which is in his commonplace book. The disease became epidemic. Deaths from it number 1021. Dr. Emerson had charge of the Hospital for Orphans. As a token of appreciation of his service during the epidemic, a silver pitcher was presented to him.

He lectured in the Franklin Institute of Pennsylvania in 1833, on meteorology, and in 1834, he delivered another course on heat, electricity and galvanism, in connection with the subject.

Dr. Emerson was chosen to be a member of the American Philosophical Society, April 19, 1833. At stated meetings he made many brief communications on many subjects, which are recorded in Vol. I to Vol. XVI of the published Proceedings. He was one of the Councilors of the Society during ten years, from 1837 till the end of 1846.

Although attentive to whatever related to agricultural improvements, he was seriously interested in medical affairs. In 1845 the New York State Medical Society invited the medical institutions of the country to appoint delegates to meet in the city of New York on the first Tuesday of May, 1846, and form a National Medical Convention to devise measures to promote the common interests of the medical profession and improve medical education. Many prominent physicians, representing medical bodies in different part of the United States, were present. Dr. Emerson, one of the delegates from the Philadelphia Society, was with them. On organizing the meeting it was found that 133 delegates from medical societies in sixteen of the twenty-nine States were duly accredited, and that seventy-five of them were from New York. This partial and unequal representation led a delegate to propose that the Convention should at once adjourn sine die. His proposition was not accepted. After due deliberation officers were elected, and committees were appointed to prepare a plan of organization, etc., and among them a committee to prepare a code of medical ethics to govern the medical profession of the United States. Dr. Emerson was appointed a member of it.

The several committees were instructed to report at a meeting of the Convention to be held on the first Wednesday of May, 1847, in Philadelphia. The National Medical Convention met at the appointed time, May 5. Of 239 delegates elected to it from twenty-two States, including the District of Columbia, 175 were present. The committees appointed in New York presented their reports, which were duly considered. The Convention, by a resolution adopted May 7, became the American Medical Association. The new organization elected officers, appointed standing committees and adjourned to meet in Baltimore on the first Tuesday of May, 1848. Dr. Emerson participated in the creation of the American Medical Association. In a note written by him on the cover of a copy of it, he claims that the Code of Medical Ethics was compiled exclusively by Dr. Isaac Hays and himself. The Association still holds its annual meetings, always to the advantage of the medical profession, and is recognized as authority on questions of medical policy in the United States. Dr. Emerson was a member of its first Committee on Publication, 1847, and served on till 1853; of the Committee on Medical Sciences, and contributed to its report of 1850, Vol. III, pp. 91-94, "Observations on Vital Statistics;" of the Committee on Hygiene, 1851; and of the Committee of Arrangements, 1855.

Dr. Emerson was elected a fellow of the College of Physicians of Philadelphia, February, 1847. He never contributed to its Transactions. He was elected a delegate from the College to the American Medical Association in 1849, and in 1858; and to the National Quarantine and Sanitary Convention in 1857, and 1858. He was a member of the Academy of Natural Sciences of Philadelphia from August, 1858; of the Philadelphia County Medical Society from 1857, of which he was President; and of the Medical Society of the State of Pennsylvania.

Dr. Emerson's medical practice from about 1828 to 1840 was lucrative and extensive. His interest in agricultural affairs, always notable, gradually increased with the lapse of time, and his interest in medical affairs gradually abated till he relinquished the practice about the year 1857.

He died very suddenly in his office, July 2, 1873, near the end of the 79th year of age. He bequeathed his ample estate, including several farms, which together contain more than a thousand acres of arable land in Delaware, to his kinsmen. His long life was virtuously spent, and so far he was above the bulk of mankind. Seemingly always under the influence of his early Quaker training by his mother, never manifesting the least pretension to piety, or solicitude about his future existence, his daily conduct was shaped in obedience to the precepts of the Decalogue and of Christianity. Naturally modest and considerate of the rights of others, he was never aggressive. A dignified and courteous demeanor, varied attainments and the easy flow of his conversation made him a welcome and frequent guest in the society of good and cultivated people.

A genius for persistent labor never permitted his talents, which were far above the average, to be idle. His career was marked by habitual industry and useful work rather than by special achievement in any of his pursuits. Though not a discoverer, or a great leader in science, his exemplary conduct and benevolent labors entitle him to general approbation, and his memory to our kindly respect.

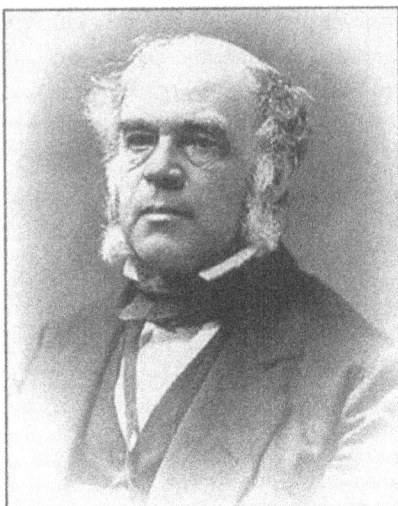

JOHN W. DRAPER

1811–1882 (APS 1844)

Memoir by William A. Hammond

In the death of Dr. Draper, the American Philosophical Society has to regret the loss of one of its most distinguished members. He died at his residence at Hastings-on-the Hudson, in the State of New York, on the fourth day of January, 1882, after an illness which had lasted with more or less severity for several months. John William Draper was born at St. Helen's, England, May 5th, 1811. His early education was received at the Wesleyan School at Woodhouse Grove, and subsequently from private teachers. At a still later period he made especial study of Chemistry, Natural Philosophy and the higher Mathematics, taking high rank in the knowledge of these sciences.

In 1833 he came to the United States, intending to make it his permanent home. Here he seems to have had his attention for the first time turned to the profession of Medicine, for he entered the Medical Department of the University of Pennsylvania and graduated in 1836. He never practised medicine, however; probably he never had a patient. A few months after receiving his diploma, he was appointed Professor of Chemistry, Physiology and Natural Philosophy in Hampden-Sidney College, in Virginia. He occupied this position for about three years, publishing during that period several important essays on chemical and physiological subjects. Some of these appeared in the American Journal of Medical Sciences, but the greater number in the London, Edinburgh and Dublin Philosophical Magazine.

In 1839 he resigned his professorship at Hampden-Sidney College, to accept that of Chemistry and Natural Philosophy in the newly inaugurated University of the City of New York. In 1841 on the origination of the Medical Department of the University, of which he was one of the founders, he was appointed Professor of Chemistry. In 1850 Physiology was combined with Chemistry and he held the joint chair. The union was continued until 1865, when Dr. Draper gave up the teaching of Chemistry in the Medical Department, continuing, however, to lecture on Physiology. In 1867 he resigned this professorship also, retaining, however, the Presidency of the Medical Faculty, which he had held from 1850. In 1873 he severed his connection altogether with the Medical Department, but continued to the day of his death to hold his professorship in the Department of Arts.

Dr. Draper was, early in his career, an experimenter in various departments of Natural Science. In 1840 he described the figures which are formed when coins are laid on polished glass and which are made visible by exposure to the action of a vapor. About the same time he began to interest himself in the discoveries being made by Daguerre and was the first to photograph the human face.

The chemical action of light was a favorite study with him. In 1844 he published his work on the "Forces which produced the Organization of Plants," in which he showed that the yellow ray of the solar spectrum is the most powerful in its influence over vegetation. One of the most important contributions made by him to science is that in which he demonstrates that all solid substances become incandescent at about the temperature of 977°F.

Dr. Draper did not confine his studies to the Natural Sciences strictly so-called. He was ambitious of distinction as a historian. His basis was, that nations are subject to the same laws as individuals and that in their migrations and stages of development they have been acted upon by purely physical causes. We are inclined to think that he carried his views in this respect, too far, and that he disregarded the undoubted influence of intellectual and emotional factors as creators and modifiers of history.

Dr. Draper's contributions to Scientific Periodicals and the Transactions of Medical Societies have been very numerous. One paper only was presented to the American Philosophical Society, and this was May 27th, 1843. He was elected a member of the Society January 19th, 1844, and consequently this memoir was submitted before he joined us: its title is, "On the Decomposition of Carbonic Acid and the Alkaline Carbonates by the Light of the Sun." It is published in Vol. III of the Proceedings.

His published volumes are as follows:
"A Treatise on the Forces which produce the Organization of Plants," 1844.
"A Text-Book of Chemistry," 1846.
"A Text-Book of Natural Philosophy," 1847.
"A Treatise of Human Physiology," 1856.
"History of the Intellectual Development of Europe," 1862.
"Thoughts on the Future Civil Policy of America," 1865.
"History of the American Civil War," 1867-70.
"History of the Conflict between Religion and Science," 1877.

In all these works Dr. Draper showed that he had read extensively and thought deeply. He had great facility for expressing himself with clearness and directness and hence for impressing his views upon others. Nevertheless it must be confessed that his chief claim for distinction will rest upon his labors in Chemistry and Natural Philosophy. His "Treatise on Human Physiology" is in many respects fanciful and speculative, and theories are promulgated as well-founded which have no support from facts. His historical works are characterized by an entire absence of references to the sources of his information, and therefore they lost much of the value which they would otherwise possess for students.

In 1876 he was awarded the Rumford Medal by the American Academy of Arts and Sciences, for his researches on Radiant Energy. In 1881 he was elected one of the twelve honorary members of the Physical Society of London.

EDITORS' NOTE

General Hammond's memoir falls short of capturing the versatility of Dr. Draper's interests and accomplishments which were unusually broad even for APS members of his time. He was a physician, scientist, astronomer, philosopher, chemist, botanist, historian and photographer. By inventing his own camera and improving on Louis Daguerre's process he took the first photograph of a human face. Through a telescope he took the first detailed photograph of the moon. He wrote papers on radiant energy, capillary attraction, respiration, the nature of flames and the condition of the sun's surface. He was a founder and for 23 years president of NYU School of Medicine. His book, "History of the Conflict Between Religion and Science" received worldwide recognition and was banned by the Catholic Church. In 1876 he became the first President of the American Chemical Society. One hundred years later NYU named its Interdisciplinary Masters Program for him.

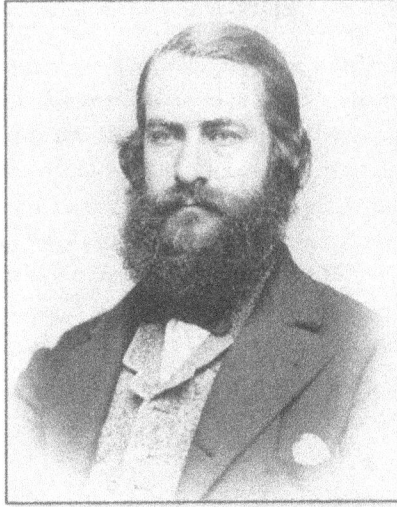

Joseph Leidy

1823–1891 (APS 1849)

Memoir by W.S.W. Ruschenberger, M.D.

In the death of Joseph Leidy, which occurred April 30, 1891 at the age of sixty-eight years, the medical profession in America lost its most loved and honored member, and American science lost its most illustrious representative. Ever modest, Dr. Leidy once introduced himself to a meeting as follows: "My name is Joseph Leidy, Doctor of Medicine. I was born in this city on the 9th of September, 1823, and I have lived here ever since. My father was Philip Leidy, the hatter on Third street above Vine. My mother was Catherine Mellick, but she died a few months after my birth. My father married her sister, Christiana Mellick, and she was a mother I have known, who was all in all to me, the one to whom I owe all that I am. At an early age I took great delight in natural history and in noticing all natural objects. I have reason to think that I know a little of natural history."

Joseph at the age of about ten years, was sent to the Classical Academy, a private day-school conducted by the Rev. William Mann, a Methodist clergyman. There he studied English and read Latin—the principal being scrupulously careful that his pupils should understand the grammar. Probably he began Greek also. Minerals and plants interested him at an early age. One day an itinerant lecturer from the so-called "universal Lyceum" visited the school, and by permission, discoursed about mineralogy, illustrating his lesson with specimens. Young Leidy was so much interested that soon after he procured books on mineralogy and botany and diligently studied them. At length he became so fascinated in the pursuit that he often absented himself from school without leave to seek specimens in the rural districts near the city. His favorite hunting ground was along the banks of the Schuylkill and Wissahickon.

Essay edited by APS Executive Officer Keith Thomson

His deep interest in mineralogy was continuous from boyhood till the close of his life. To him it was a kind of Sunday afternoon or holiday recreation to visit friends who had cabinets, examine their newly acquired specimens and talk about them in connection with those in rival collections. Always seeking to obtain rare specimens, especially of gems he bought and sold, he exchanged minerals with his friends whenever opportunity occurred. He continually added to and improved his cabinet which, at his death was sold to the National Museum at Washington, DC for $2800.

He had manifested at an early age uncommon aptitude in draughting and drawing; his father conjectured that he would succeed as a sign painter. But the son, who had passed much of his leisure in the wholesale drug store of his cousin, Napoleon B. Leidy, M.D., "physician and druggist," as the City Directory styled him, fancied that he would rather be an apothecary. His loving stepmother, however, was not satisfied. She seemed sure that there was in him the making of a successful physician. In the autumn of 1840, he became a pupil of Dr. James McClintock, then a private teacher of anatomy in College avenue. Leidy matriculated the University of Pennsylvania, October 6, 1841, and was under the instruction of Dr. Paul B. Goddard, then Demonstrator of Anatomy in the University. Having attended three courses of lectures and submitted a thesis on The comparative anatomy of the eye of vertebrated animals, the degree of Doctor of Medicine was conferred upon him April 4, 1844 by the University of Pennsylvania.

In the autumn he opened an office, No. 211 North Sixth street, hoping to obtain employment as a general practitioner. But the business which came to him during two years' trial did not promise a satisfactory living, and therefore he determined to devote himself exclusively to teaching. Possibly his failure to obtain practice was ascribable in some degree to lack of due attention to patients. Years after this time, to show how intently attractive comparative anatomy was to him, he related to his private class that on one occasion he was so absorbed in his office studying the anatomy of a work that he totally forgot that he had to be called to an obstetric case which he had engaged to attend.

In 1845, the Professor of Anatomy, Dr. Horner, appointed Dr. Leidy his prosector. In 1846 he was chosen Demonstrator of Anatomy in the Franklin Medical College, but resigned the office at the close of the session and, in 1847, resumed his position with Dr. Horner and delivered to his students a private course of lectures on Human Anatomy. In the spring of 1848, impaired health induced Prof. Horner to visit Europe. He invited his friend, Dr. Leidy, to be his traveling companion. They sailed in April and returned in September. In England, Germany and France they "visited hospitals and anatomical museums and sought out eminent anatomists and surgeons." Dr. Leidy witnessed in Paris, June 20, some vivisection experiments by Magendie, in his physiological laboratory, which interested him. They "were in Vienna while the revolutionary movements were in progress:" and "were also in Paris during the fierce conflicts from 23nd to 26th of June; and during several days afterwards they "witnessed in the hospitals, filled with wounded, every variety of gunshot wound and the modes of treatment pursued."

On his return from Europe, in the autumn, Dr. Leidy delivered a course of lectures on Microscopic Anatomy; and in the sprint of 1849 began a course on Physiology in the Medical Institute of Philadelphia, which the condition of his health required him to abandon. An interesting event enabled Dr. Leidy to go abroad again under very favorable circumstances. Dr. George B. Wood, who was elected May, 1850, Professor of the Practice of Medicine desired to collect in Europe models, casts, preparations, etc., suitable for objective illustration of his future courses of instruction. Aware of the artistic judgment of Dr. Leidy, and of his recently acquired knowledge of localities in which objects adapted to his purpose could be purchased, Dr. Wood easily persuaded him to be his companion and assistant in hunting and selecting desirable specimens.

Dr. Leidy was elected a Fellow of the College of Physicians of Philadelphia, August 1851. He was Secretary of the Committee on Lectures under the Mütter Trust, from January 1864. He lectured on Physiology in the Medical Institute of Philadelphia in the summer courses of 1851 and 1852. In May Dr. Leidy was elected Professor of Anatomy. He was yet in the thirtieth year of his age. On nomination by Dr. Samuel George Morton and Messrs. John S. Phillips and John Cassin, Dr. Leidy was elected a member of the Academy of Natural Sciences of Philadelphia, July 29, 1845.

Dr. Leidy's first important work in natural history was begun in the winter of 1844, at the instance of Mr. Amos Binney, President of the Boston Society of Natural History. It is entitled *Special Anatomy of the Terrestrial Gasteropoda of the United States*. In 1847 Dr. Leidy made a discovery concerning the parasitic worm Trichina spiralis which commonly infests humans. It had been described in England by Richard Owen in 1835. No one had ever suggested a source of or how this parasite found its way into the human subject until Dr. Leidy, while eating a piece of ham at his own breakfast table, discovered its existence in the hog. The discovery that Trichina spiralis infests the hog is, in its economic relations, among the most important observations Dr. Leidy every made. One consequence was that the importation of American pork to Europe was banned until it was established that thorough cooking renders trichinous pork harmless.

Dr. Leidy was chosen a member of the American Philosophical Society October 19, 1849. Though not frequently present at its meetings, he contributed several papers to its Transactions and Proceedings. The University of Pennsylvania appointed Dr. Leidy its delegate to the American Medical Association in 1854 at St. Louis, Mo., and in 1872 at Philadelphia. Dr. Leidy was on the list of permanent members of the Association from 1854 to 1876. At the St. Louis meeting he was appointed Chairman of a Committee on Diseases of Parasitic Origin. The Committees of the Association on Medical Literature and on Medical Science cited with encomium his papers, *On the Comparative Structure of the Liver*, *On the Intermaxillary Bone in the Embryo of the Human Subject*, and *On Parasitic Life*.

Dr. Leidy continued to teach anatomy and to conduct microscopical work, with a special interest in both the symbiotic and parasitic animals of vertebrates. In 1851, he published an extensive memoir on *A Flora and Fauna within Living Animals*, but by this time his work had taken a new and perhaps surprising direction. In 1841 the great British geologist Charles Lyell visited American and went to meet Leidy whose anatomical skill and meticulous drawings had already made him famous. He advised Leidy to turn to paleontology. "Don't bother with medicine. Stick to paleontology. That is your future."

Microscopic anatomy was not entirely without its charms, however. In 1846 Napolean Leidy, his cousin, asked for forensic help in a murder case, in which the defendant claimed that the incriminating blood on his clothing was from a chicken. Leidy easily showed that it was human blood because human red blood cells are easily identified microscopically by their lack of a nucleus.

Five years after Lyell's visit, Leidy made his first description of a fossil and typically, it was a significant discovery—the teeth of the first fossil horse from North America. This was the time when the American West was being first closely explored and ranchers and traders began sending to Leidy fossils of a wide array of extinct mammals. One of the earliest new genera for Leidy to name was

Paleotherium. Many valuable specimens came from the Oligocene badlands between the White River and the Black Hills and over the next two decades the trickle of exciting material entirely new to science became a flood. He even described, under another name, the first fossil of the dinosaur Tyrannosaurus.

One of the most important fossil vertebrate associated with Leidy, who in 1858 helped dig it up, studied it, and named it was Hadrosaurus foulki, from nearby Haddonfield, N.J. This was the first discovery and description of an articulated skeleton of a dinosaur. Eventually the specimen was assembled in a life-like pose by the English artist Waterhouse Hawkins (who had created the displays of dinosaur models at London's Crystal Palace exhibits). It was put on display at the Academy of Natural Sciences. So many people came to see the dinosaur that admissions charges had to be instituted.

Leidy was an extremely modest man, avoiding the limelight in his private and scientific life, and eschewing theory in favor of the simple presentation of facts. With Hadrosaurus, however, he made a vital contribution to palaeontological theory in realizing that the animal had been bipedal, standing on its hind legs and that helped confirm the idea of Thomas Henry Huxley that dinosaurs were related to birds – now the orthodox view. He accepted, without reserve, all the theories of evolution, etc., of Mr. Darwin, with whom he had correspondence, but their religious views were very different.

In 1861 he published An Elementary Treatise on Human Anatomy, and in 1889, the work having been out of print many years, a second edition, rewritten and enlarged. The illustrations are largely from his own drawings of many recent dissections made by him in connection with this work. In 1862, when the "Satterlee," a U.S. Army Hospital, was established in West Philadelphia, Dr. Leidy was assigned the task of conducting the autopsies and reporting them, from time to time, to the Surgeon-General of the Army. Dr. Joseph Leidy was appointed a member of the Sanitary Commission Association, April 3, 1862.

In August, 1864, Dr. Leidy married Anna, a daughter of Robert Harden, of Louisville, Ky. To compensate for the sterility of this union, they some years afterwards adopted the infant daughter of a deceased friend. Dr. Leidy told the writer that had this dear child been his own he could not have loved her more.

About the year 1866 it was suggested that natural history should be taught in the University. The proposition was entertained and discussed from time to time, and lingered on without action.

Dr. Leidy was appointed for the current academic year, Professor of Biology (Zoölogy) in the Faculty of Philosophy. In 1884 the department was organized by the appointment of a Faculty of seven professors, including Dr. Leidy as Professor of Zoölogy and Comparative Anatomy, and he was elected, May 6, Director of the Biological Department.

Both before and after the War between the States, Leidy conducted his researches on Western fossils from his laboratory in Philadelphia, leaving the young geologist Ferdinand Vandeveer Hayden (subsequently professor of Geology at the University of Pennsylvania) to act as his alter ego and agent in the west. Meanwhile Leidy's protégé Edward Drinker Cope in Philadelphia and Othniel Charles Marsh at Harvard had begun vying for the popularity or notoriety attached to the discovery of fossils from the west. They traveled out west themselves, trying beat each other to the best specimens, essentially "poaching" Leidy's territory. Dr. Leidy named more than three hundred new species of fossils but not until 1871 did he venture to the West for himself and by then he had essentially given up the subject. He had neither the stomach not the necessary deep pockets to compete in a rivalry that had come to range geographically over the entire country. While Cope and Marsh were working the fossiliferous field into which Dr Leidy had entered long before, and by his labor made, in a sense, his own, they fell into disputes over priority of dates of different names of genera and species found in the later strata of a Western territory, in which contention Leidy, the friend of both, refused to take any part. So dominant was his repugnance to controversy of any kind that he left his friends, freed from his participation and for a considerable period engaged in an entirely different field of investigation, to return long afterwards to his beloved paleontology.

The ill-feeling that grew up between Leidy and Cope was exacerbated on the occasion when Marsh came to Philadelphia to examine the skeleton of an enormous marine reptile called Elasmosaurus that Cope had described. Marsh saw instantly that Cope had reconstructed it with the head on the wrong end. Leidy was called into the laboratory at the Academy of Natural Sciences to adjudicate. He silently picked up the head, put in on the proper end, and, without uncharacteristic coldness, left the room.

Dr. Leidy returned to the quiet of the laboratory and to his microscope. Of the two summers that he spent exploring the country around Fort Bridger, the Uinta mountains and Salt Lake basin, he was mostly engaged in search of materials for his great treatise on Fresh Water Rhizopods of North America, under the auspices of the U.S. Geological and Geographical Survey of the Territories, then directed by Dr. Hayden. The work was published in 1879.

He passed the summer of 1875 in Europe, visiting museums in London, Paris, Berlin and mingling socially with renowned professors and distinguished votaries of natural science where he halted. The Boston Society of Natural History, January 22, 1880, "Voted that the Walker Grand Honorary Prize for 1879 be awarded to Prof. Joseph Leidy for his prolonged investigations and discoveries in zoology and paleontology and in consideration of their extraordinary merit the sum awarded be $1000. In December 1881, he was elected without competition President of the Academy of Natural Sciences of Philadelphia, and continuously held the office till he died.

The Trustees of the Wagner Free Institute of Science elected him, July 27, 1885, President of the Faculty and Professor of Biology, at an annual salary of $500. From that date the Trustees obtained his views before deciding any question relating to the scientific policy of the Institute, and appointed members of the Faculty subject to his approval. He lectured two or three times every season, and always attracted a large audience. At the summer commencement of 1886, Harvard University conferred upon him its honorary degree of Legum Doctor—LL.D.; and the Institute of France awarded to him, December 18, 1888, the Cuvier prize medal.

Because of his gentle manner and dislike of controversy, Dr. Leidy was one of the most beloved Philadelphians. It may be truly said that he was born to be a naturalist. To his innate ability to perceive the minutest variations in the forms and color of things was united artistic aptitude of a high order. These natural faculties, in continuous exercise almost from his infantile days, and his love of accuracy, enabled him to detect minute difference and resemblances of all objects, and to correctly describe and portray them. Besides, nothing, however small, that came within the scope of his vision, while walking or riding, escaped his notice.

Dr. Leidy had a rare experience of living nearly sixty-eight years without provoking personal hostility, without making an enemy. Troops of friends encouraged his pursuits, and among them some were ever ready to give him, when needed, substantial help to publish his works. No votary of natural history was helped more or more favored or more popular.

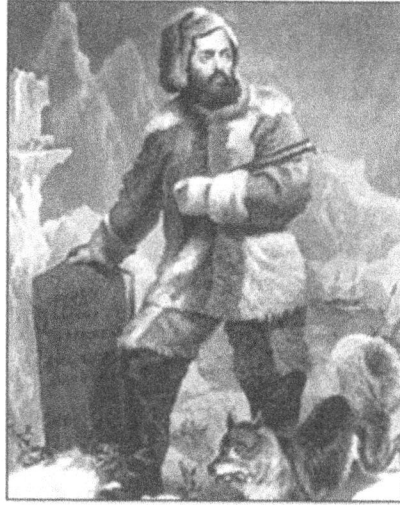

ELISHA KENT KANE
1820–1856 (APS 1851)
Memoir by APS Library staff

Whether because of—or in spite of—a debilitating childhood bout with rheumatic fever that left him with a delicate constitution, Elisha Kent Kane went on to live an adventurous life and "die in the harness," as his father had wished. Each of the half-dozen brilliant forays that he made into the exotic seems to have been terminated by accident or illness, but from these experiences, Kane carefully built a public image for himself as America's great tragic hero of exploration.

Elisha Kent Kane was born in Philadelphia on February 3, 1820, the son of the jurist and Democratic politician John Kintzing Kane and his wife Jane Duval Leiper. Already prominent in Philadelphia and Washington, the Kane family became more so with Elisha's celebrity as an Arctic explorer and his brother, Thomas Leiper Kane's, as a general in the Union army and advocate for the Mormons.

Upon first entering college at the University of Virginia, Elisha intended to study geology and civil engineering, but on the advice of family friends, he transferred to the University of Pennsylvania to take up medicine, graduating in 1842. With receipt of his degree, however, his concerned family members believed that a medical practice might be too rigorous for the frail young man, and they sought to discourage him from the profession. But unbeknownst to Elisha, his father arranged a surgeon's commission in the navy, and upon graduation, Elisha was directed to report to the Philadelphia Navy Yard to be examined for assignment. Despite his medical history, Kane passed the examination and received his commission in the following year.

In his first assignment, Kane joined the diplomat Caleb Cushing on the first American diplomatic mission to China in May 1843. The voyage to the Far East was the first of many adventures for Kane, which included a daring descent into a Philippine volcano, apparently inciting controversy among locals. At the completion of trade negotiations in June 1844, Kane resigned from the Cushing Commission and elected to remain in China for six months, operating a hospital boat with a young English surgeon. Although the venture was successful financially, Kane contracted cholera and was forced to abandon his practice and return home. By the time that he reached Philadelphia in the summer of 1845, he had logged thousands of miles and visited five continents.

Despite his stated intentions of settling down and opening a medical practice in the city, Kane soon enlisted for another tour of duty at sea, this time taking a cruise to Africa aboard the frigate *United States*. It has been suggested that Kane's precipitous decision to ship out had less to do with a thirst for adventure than it did a taste of scandal. Shortly after his return to Philadelphia Kane had begun spending time with a young woman named Julia Reed, and several months later, he was scurrying to conceal her pregnancy. While historian and Kane biographer George W. Conner (APS Executive Officer 1960–1977) acknowledged that there was some correspondence to support the basis for the scandal, he nevertheless maintained that an out of wedlock pregnancy "did not fit" Kane's gentlemanly character. Regardless of the circumstances, however, sail away Kane did in May 1846, leaving behind a despondent family and two heartbroken cousins, Mary Leiper and Helen Patterson. Although Kane did not appear to enjoy his African sojourn, it afforded him the opportunity to study the slave trade at first hand, a topic of great interest to the Kane family, and especially to his abolitionist brother Thomas and to his father.

Just as in China, however, illness cut short Kane's cruise, and he returned home weak, emaciated, and depressed, and just as in China, he was not held back for long. Even before he had recovered from his bout of "coast fever," he traveled to Washington to petition for a transfer into the army in order to fight in the Mexican War. The prospects of escape and adventure and of military glory were always supremely attractive to Kane, but after contracting yet another debilitating illness, he gave up hope of active duty. Failing in his attempt to sign on as physician to Girard College, he renewed his push for a transfer, and when President James Polk decided he needed a messenger to relay information to General Winfield Scott, Kane was offered the assignment.

En route to Mexico, Kane wrote to his father to assure him that the "Philadelphia Kane family is represented in the war," and he challenged him to use this "representation" to further advance the Kane family. Ultimately, Kane's stint in the army did bring credit to his family's name. Wounded in a battle with Mexican forces, Kane distinguished himself by saving the life of Mexican General Antonio Gaona, and in return, Gaona and his family nursed Kane back to health in their luxurious compound after the illness-prone Philadelphian had fallen ill with "congestive typhus fever." Declared unfit for further duty, Kane was sent home to a hero's welcome.

After a slow convalescence over the summer, Kane unsuccessfully applied for a position at the Philadelphia Navy Yard, and then for an assignment aboard the store ship *Supply*, scheduled to sail for Lisbon, the Mediterranean, and Rio de Janeiro. Reminiscent in many ways of Kane's African trip, the *Supply* cruise was uneventful apart from the brutal floggings meted out frequently on the backs of the unruly crew that Kane, as ship's surgeon, was obligated to attend. In September 1849, Kane left his assignment aboard the *Supply*, and signed on aboard the surveying steamer *Walker*, bound for Mobile Bay on coastguard service.

While the experience aboard the *Supply* deepened Kane's aversion to shipboard brutality, he found his coastguard duty irredeemably dull. Kane yearned for adventure, and early in the following year, the perfect opportunity presented itself: a rescue expedition was forming to search for the lost explorer Sir

John Franklin, who had last been seen on July 22, 1845 en route to locate a Northwest Passage to the Pacific Ocean.

On May 22, 1850, Kane set sail aboard the brig *Advance*, one of two ships supplied for the expedition by the whaling magnate Henry Grinnell. The U.S. Navy crew under the command of Lieutenant Edwin De Haven, was charged with searching for Franklin in Baffin Bay, but he was ordered thereafter to proceed northward in search of the still undiscovered Northwest Passage. There were ten other rescue ships in the Arctic that summer. Between August 25th and 27th, the crews of Captain John Penny and De Haven landed on the shores of Cape Riley where they discovered evidence of an encampment, presumably Franklin's, and additional evidence was discovered on Beechey Island, ten miles further up Wellington Channel. Since Franklin had left no indication of the direction in which he was headed, the captains agreed to split up and continue their search over a wider area, with De Haven heading north up Wellington Channel.

In early September, the *Advance* passed Cornwallis Island and began heading further north before it was stopped altogether by a howling storm. Scrubbing the mission, De Haven elected to try to return home, but as ice formed around the ships and locked them into a floe, they found themselves trapped, and pushed steadily northward. Even when the floe broke up temporarily, the ship was freed only long enough to become frozen into another icepack headed south. By October 1st, Kane and his shipmates realized that they faced a winter in the Arctic.

In the dark and bitterly cold winter, De Haven and many in the crew became desperately ill with scurvy, leaving their health and survival in Dr. Kane's hands. Ordering them to exercise, even on the coldest days, and increasing their rations, Kane is credited with saving their lives. After having been pushed out of Wellington Channel, eastward through Lancaster Sound, and southward down Baffin Bay, the ship was finally freed of the ice on June 5, 1851, and was able to make its way to Greenland's Disco Island to replenish stores for another season of exploration.

From Upernavik, the expedition set sail again in early July and soon after hit solid ice. By mid-August, the frustrated De Haven abandoned the mission and headed for New York before facing another arctic winter. Although they had failed to locate Franklin or the Northwest Passage, when Kane returned home, he was once again received as a hero.

Making the most of the acclaim, Kane spent the next year traveling and lecturing on his Arctic adventures to capacity crowds. His celebrity grew enormously as a result of his colorful lectures, and carefully edited accounts of his Arctic adventures filled the newspapers. Perhaps most famously, he worked tirelessly to promote his theory that Franklin had drifted into a warm-water Open Polar Sea that he was sure circled the pole. Using the attention resulting from his book, *The U. S. Grinnell Expedition in Search of Sir John Franklin*, Kane raised funds for a second expedition, taking the largest share from the magnanimous Henry Grinnell, who agreed to once again offer use of the *Advance*. It appeared as though Kane would have every opportunity to test his theory.

The fall of 1852 was marked by two significant events: the tragic death of fourteen year-old Willie Kane and the introduction of Elisha Kent Kane to Margaret Fox, one the best known Spiritualist mediums in America. Willie's death devastated the entire family, so much so that they abandoned their mansion on the outskirts of Philadelphia and moved back into the city, unable to bear living in Willie's house any longer. Elisha, who had kept watch at Willie's bedside for several weeks, was particularly affected. There has been some speculation that Kane's grief led him to seek out the comfort of Spiritualist communication with the dead; however, there is no evidence that Kane ever actually discussed

Willie with Maggie Fox. Nevertheless, after several visits to the hotel where Fox held seances, Kane's spirits improved, and as he labored to finish his book and to complete organization for his expedition, he continued to pay regular visits.

Although their relationship started out casually, Kane began to make demands on Fox. Initially unconcerned over the propriety of her "calling," he soon began to urge her to give it up, and at the same time, he began to insist that she become more ladylike, proposing that she allow him to send her to school. For her part, Fox seemed uncertain whether she would comply or resist, but as their relationship grew more intense, the demands became more important. At one point, Kane broke off the relationship, recognizing that one of them would have to give up their "cause," something that neither was willing to do.

Fox must have had a change of heart, because a few months later she wrote to Kane expressing dissatisfaction with her "very tiresome life" and asking his advice. His immediate reply encouraged her to "stick to your good resolutions" and reaffirmed his commitment to helping her escape a life which, according to Kane, was "worse than tedious, it is sinful." Maggie's mother finally agreed to allow Kane to arrange for Maggie's education, and the Turner family of rural Crookville, Pennsylvania, was engaged to provide board for Maggie while she attended school nearby. Kane also made arrangements with Cornelius Grinnell to pay her board and take care of other incidental expenses. The young couple agreed that if Kane was sufficiently satisfied with Fox's reeducation when he returned from the Arctic, they would be married, but until then they could not become engaged. On May 27, 1853, Fox moved into the Turner's home in Crookville, and four days later Kane departed for the Arctic.

From the beginning, Kane was concerned that news of his relationship with Fox could harm his reputation while he was away, so he enlisted the help of Cornelius Grinnell and younger brother Robert Patterson Kane to help safeguard Elisha's reputation. Patterson and Grinnell were to act as couriers for correspondence between Fox and Kane and they were instructed to quell any rumors that arose. Kane left his correspondence regarding his role in Maggie's education with his brother in order to leave a paper trail indicating that he was nothing more than a generous benefactor of the young woman.

There were other matters to worry about as well—Kane's health, as usual, among them. In April 1853, just one month prior to sailing, Kane was stricken with rheumatic fever, but even after being confined to bed for three weeks, unsure whether he might die, he decided that he would make a go of the expedition. Such an unpromising beginning was a sign of things to come. The usual bouts of seasickness and an inexperienced crew added to the concerns, but it was only when the expedition reached the Arctic that the real troubles began.

Already concerned that he might be trumped in the discovery of the Open Polar Sea, Kane grew frantic upon receiving a letters from Lady Jane Franklin informing him that Capt. Edward Inglefield was setting out in one of England's best steam-powered ships to follow the rescue path that Kane had pursued in 1850-1851. Although Inglefield had only been sent to the Arctic to deliver supplies to five ships on Beechey Island, Lady Franklin's letter led Kane to adopt a more aggressive course than he had originally planned, crossing directly through Mellville Bay. Although this route stood to save time, it would expose the ship to treacherous icebergs which blocked the entrances to Smith and Lancaster Sounds, and Kane recognized that by taking this course he would also risk being frozen into an ice floe for the winter. He decided to take the chance.

Ominously, while crossing Mellville Bay, the *Advance* suffered a head-on collision with an iceberg that destroyed the jig-boom and one of the lifeboats, yet the ship still made remarkable time. By early

August, with the entrance to Smith Sound in sight, the *Advance* stopped at Littleton Island to leave provisions and a lifeboat for future emergencies before pushing northward, and it was there that their troubles really began. Facing lashing storms and ice-clogged waters, Kane ultimately had to order his men to strap themselves into harnesses and pull the ship north. By late August, the *Advance* had traveled further north than any previous expedition (by the American route), but Kane demanded they push still further. But when the crew protested—and more importantly, when it was ascertained that no further progress could be made due to heavy ice—Kane agreed that they should stay put and wait for spring. While the American public waited and worried, Kane and his crew settled in for the winter.

The crew prepared for winter by building supply houses on shore, a wooden cover for the ship's deck, and a kennel for the dogs. Repeated attempts to rid themselves of the ship's rat population were somewhat successful but the methods caused a few anxious moments. The first attempt using noxious fumes nearly killed the cook, and the second, asphyxiation by carbon monoxide, set the deck on fire and caused Kane and another crew member to lose consciousness while battling the blaze.

By mid-October, when the sun disappeared, all activity ground to a halt, and Kane and his crew were confined below deck to ride out a harsh winter ridden with scurvy and sensory deprivation, and more than a few flares of temper and fist fights. By February, with the sun barely visible, Kane wasted no time in returning to the mission, selecting eight members of the crew to attempt to reach Humboldt glacier and beyond. Ignoring the bitter cold and the protests of the experienced crew members that it was still too early to proceed, he sent his squad northward in mid-March.

The attempt was short-lived. Within a week of their departure, three of the men stumbled back to ship with news that the others were ill and freezing. Kane immediately led a party to rescue the men, an excursion that took fifty hours in temperatures that fell at times to fifty below zero. At the same time, the crew spied several Inuit hunters from Etah, a small village just 70 miles to the south, and invited them on board, where they sat down to a meal of raw walrus that the Inuit had brought with them. With the help of Carl Christian Peterson, a Danish crew member fluent in Inuktitut, Kane was able to communicate with the Inuit, enlisting their help for the upcoming winter.

As spring approached, Kane began to implement his plan to head north in search of the Open Polar Sea. First, he intended to send six of his men by foot to Humboldt Glacier, with him and another crew member following on a sledge with provisions. They would then cross the channel to the American side and search for openings to the Open Polar Sea. As May—and warmer weather—approached, Kane realized that if he was to make a move, it would have to be before rising temperatures melted the ice. Yet once again, nothing went quite right. Heavy snowdrifts and the effects of scurvy and snow-blindness stalled the expedition, and the crew discovered that all the food they had cached during the previous fall had been eaten by polar bears. Eventually, though, a small party from Kane's crew made it to Humboldt Glacier and crossed the still-frozen "Kane Basin." Despite battling snow blindness, they managed to travel over two hundred miles in all. Within a week of the first group's return to the ship, Kane sent out a second party of six men to travel beyond Humboldt Glacier to see if they could verify the existence of an opening to the Open Polar Sea.

On June 5, the men set off for Humboldt Glacier, two of whom continued northward after the others attempted to ascend the glacier and failed. Kane feared the worst for the two, but on July 3rd, they returned with the news that Kane had longed to hear: they had discovered the Open Polar Sea. They described how Kane Basin narrowed into a channel, and as they pressed further north, they noticed thinning ice and swarms of birds, including an open water species, the Arctic Petrel. They climbed a cape and from a 480 foot height, they saw nothing but open water. Kane was elated: having attained their goal, it looked as if he and his crew could finally focus on going home. There were only two small problems: the basin was frozen solid, completely blocking the way and the ship itself was completely iced in. It appeared that the *Advance* might face yet another Arctic winter.

Any hopes that the warm temperatures and strong winds might break up the floe were dashed when Kane discovered that new ice was already beginning to form and that the escape route was narrowing further. As August drew to a close, Kane accepted that the ship was trapped, but several members of the crew began to plan their escape. Feeling that he could not, in good conscience, force them to stay, Kane announced on August 23rd that if any men wished to strike out on their own, he would not stop them. Only five elected to stay: the others he made sign documents attesting that they were deserting and that Kane was no longer responsible for them. To his credit, Kane suppressed his anger long enough to bid the departing men good luck and to assure them that should they decide to return, they would be welcomed.

Kane and the remaining crew prepared for another Arctic winter, fortified with a year's experience and some valuable lessons in survival learned from the Inuit. Their first task was to insulate the ship to make it as "igloo-like" as possible. Although the darkness was oppressive, the relative comfort of the ship as well as the mutual hunting agreement with the people of Etah promised to make the winter months much more bearable. In early December, two deserters returned to the *Advance* and the others arrived shortly thereafter, having never made it to Upernavik. Kane suppressed his resentment and welcomed them as promised, even though sheltering the extra men proved to be a big challenge—one of several as it turned out.

The cramped living space and strain on food stores increased tensions among the men, and illness, falling temperatures, and diminishing fuel supplies added to the misery. Tempers flared along with illness and insubordination. Kane kept discipline by calling offenders up on deck individually and bashing them "in the side of the head with a heavy metal belaying pin." This, it seemed, was an effective if temporary method.

The food shortage was the most critical issue, and Kane's hopes of leaning on the generosity of the Inuit were dashed when it was discovered that the residents of Etah were starving, too. Kane arranged to combine efforts with the Inuit in hunting, and together they managed to kill a walrus, saving both groups from starvation. Discipline, however, remained an issue. Two crew members, William Godfrey and John Blake, were discovered to be planning to steal a sledge bound for Etah. Although the men were caught in time and were beaten with a "leaden fist," Godfrey managed to escape on foot. Still weak from disease and hunger, the crew suffered for two weeks before the would-be thief returned with the sledge filled with meat. Godfrey refused to board the ship even when Kane brandished a rifle and shot at him, but instead ran off. Although Kane was furious, the meat helped restore the crew's health and spirits. Godfrey later claimed that he had not deserted a second time because he had never entered into an agreement with Kane upon his return from the first secession.

As spring approached, the crew's health and morale slowly improved and preparations began for the journey home. Although Kane was disappointed that he had been unable to see the Open Polar Sea for himself, he did manage to see Humboldt Glacier. On May 20, 1855, he and his crew began pulling their whale boats (their ship having been dismantled for fuel) over the ice to open water. By mid-June they were in Etah, and after waiting out a short spell of severe weather, they bid their Inuit friends farewell and set off for Upernavik.

In a punishing journey that left one crew member dead, the small boats were pitched about violently in the ice-filled waters, and several times the men had to take cover from the heavy winds and ice. Solid ice at the base of Cape York led Kane to move out into Melville Bay instead of staying close to shore and waiting for the ice to move. By early August, however, Kane and his crew reached Upernavik, and from there they passed to Godhavn and on September 11th, met up with an American ship sent to their rescue.

When Kane arrived in New York on October 11th, 1854, he was once again accorded a hero's welcome. Advised by his family to handle his reception with humility and gratitude, he thanked the nation for their interest and concern, and much to his relief, no one on the crew sought to contradict his account of his crew's camaraderie and unity, or his own strong leadership. As it turned out, his greatest challenge lay within his own family: they were still very much opposed to his relationship with Maggie Fox.

Maggie had moved to Philadelphia in late September 1854 in anticipation of Kane's arrival, and two days later, the two were together at Clinton Place. The long-awaited reunion, however, was not the romantic encounter anticipated. Instead, Maggie found Kane to be distracted and agitated. Bowing to family pressure to cut off the relationship, he pleaded with Maggie to sign a note stating that their relationship was purely platonic. She refused. He returned a few days later with a reporter in tow, requesting that she affirm that they had never been engaged. Again, Maggie refused.

Rumors of Kane's engagement began to circulate widely, and even his departure for Washington, D.C., to give an official account of the expedition did nothing to quash them. To the family's dismay, a small newspaper in upstate New York reported the engagement, and soon major newspapers across the country were reprinting the story. Using its influence, the Kane family forced retraction of the story, but when Kane failed to refute the retraction, Maggie ended the relationship.

Nevertheless, he and Maggie continued to correspond. Kane clearly agonized over his decision but he and his family had built his public image very carefully and were not about to let a fling with a Spiritualist undo their hard work. Maggie, who had to preserve her own reputation, felt she had little choice either. Marriage, one possible solution, would preserve Maggie's reputation, but diminish the Kane family's standing—something he was unwilling or unable to do until he was financially solvent. In the meantime, Maggie, her sister Kate, and their mother moved to 22nd Street in New York.

The Navy had already given Kane permission to publish his account of his Arctic experiences and had paid him for the time it took to write it. It was a generous arrangement, perhaps because the Navy had suffered criticism for not initially supporting Kane's expedition. At any rate, Kane wasted no time in picking a publisher, George W. Childs, who also worked aggressively to promote Kane's image—so aggressively in fact, that his efforts to goad Congress into purchasing a large number of copies resulted in accusations that Kane was using his family's political connections for personal gain. Some of Child's other efforts fared better, including marketing the book at trade shows and selling it door-to-door, and Kane's public appearances also increased sales. Although the book was well-received and sold well, Kane was miserable. In addition to being unable to marry Maggie Fox, he had another problem: Lady Jane Franklin was determined that he head yet another expedition to rescue her husband.

Lady Franklin was, by all accounts, a determined advocate for her still-missing husband, and although nine years had elapsed since her husband had disappeared, she was effective at ratcheting up public pressure to save him. Kane felt obligated to lead the expedition and in August 1856, he began efforts to secure support. Kane spent the remainder of the fall (as he had the spring and summer) with

Fox at her family's New York residence. By this point, her family had come to accept Kane as a sincere suitor, and he was welcome in their home, yet because his own family continued to hold back, he took great pains to conceal the relationship. Only his brother Patterson was kept informed, and perhaps only then because Kane assured him of his discretion.

On October 11, 1856, Kane left for Liverpool, arriving in poor health after a rough crossing. His spirits must have been relatively high, because he entertained thoughts of securing funding for not one, but two expeditions, and he wrote to his parents to ask them to seek support in the United States. It was not to be. On October 29, Kane collapsed and was sent to the suburbs of London to rest. From there he traveled to Cuba to take advantage of the better climate. Kane and his steward, William Morton, left for St. Thomas on November 17, but on the voyage between St. Thomas and Cuba, Kane suffered a stroke.

Kane's brother Thomas was waiting in Havana, and was joined in mid-January by his mother, and his brother John. After a brief rally, Elisha suffered a second, more severe stroke, and on February 16, he died at the age of 37.

EDITORS' NOTE

Elisha Kent Kane was something more than just a physician, explorer and adventurer. During his lifetime he may have been the Nation's most famous person. He was America's hero! Fanciful children's books were written about his exploits. Named for him were US Navy ships, redwood trees, geographic sites and craters on the moon. George Connor (APS Executive Officer 1960–1977) in his biography of Kane asserts that Kane died from sub-acute bacterial endocarditis, an infection of his rheumatic fever damaged heart valves. As a physician Kane would have realized that he was doomed to an early death from this condition, which was incurable before antibiotics. Perhaps he even reflected that he might be protected from bacterial infection by the arctic temperatures while at increased risk on his return to warmer climates such as the Caribbean's.

When Kane died in Cuba the Nation mourned. Cuba's governor took his body to New Orleans. Its progress by boat up the Mississippi was interrupted by crowds lining the river's banks and every small town wharf. The train trip from Cincinnati to Philadelphia took four days because of the throngs on the tracks. In Philadelphia Kane's body lay in state in Independence Hall. His funeral was the largest in American history, eclipsed only by that of Abraham Lincoln a few years later.

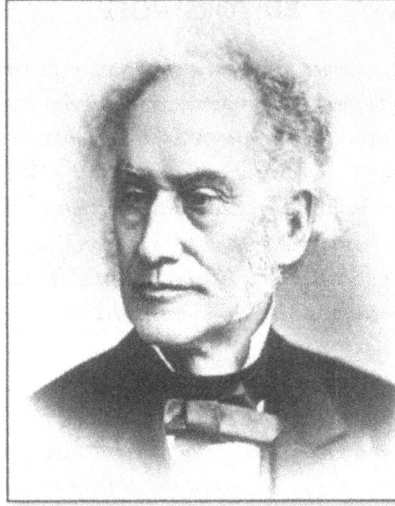

SAMUEL D. GROSS

1805–1884 (APS 1854)

Memoir by J. M. Da Costa

Samuel David Gross was born in the neighborhood of Easton, Pennsylvania, on July the 8th, 1805. At school he was an industrious boy, and he received a good education at the Wilkesbarre Academy and the Lawrenceville High School. He never went to college; but when at the age of nineteen he began to read medicine, it was evident that the young votary of science had been accustomed to intellectual labor, and was taking up his professional studies with no untrained mind.

On enrolling himself as a student at the Jefferson Medical College, of Philadelphia, he was at the same time an office pupil of Professor George McClellan, if one of the most eccentric, also one of the most original and successful surgeons of his day; and it is very likely that young Gross, who through life preserved a veneration for his brilliant preceptor, got his bias for surgery from this association.

And how he worked as a student! Tales are still current at the College, transmitted through janitors and college servitors, and losing nothing in coloring by the diffusion through the successive classes the eminent professor subsequently taught, of how immense had been his labors; how he rose with the early dawn; was never seen without a book under his arm; and had to be turned out from the anatomical rooms by the wearied attendants when the hour for closing them arrived. Certain it is he worked with his whole heart; and when he graduated in 1828 he was a noted man in his class.

He began the practice of his profession in a little office in Fourth street, in Philadelphia, and it is said that he had among the visitors who dropped in on him his future colleague, Joseph Pancoast. More friendly visitors than patients, it is to be feared, came to his rooms; for after about two years, his patrimony being nearly spent, he gave up the struggle in a great medical centre and returned to Easton.

But he carried with him evidence of his love of learning and of his indomitable perseverance. He

82

had in the short time translated from the French and the German works on General Anatomy, on Obstetrics, on Operative Surgery, and he had published his treatise on "The Anatomy, Physiology, and Diseases of the Bones and Joints." He also took away with him a wife, a lady of English descent of many accomplishments, who proved to him a true helpmate in his arduous career.

It was not long before Dr. Gross became a leading practitioner in the flourishing little town of Easton, and his scientific knowledge was so well appreciated that he was offered the Chair of Chemistry in the well-known College seated there, in Lafayette College. He declined it; but finding that within him which impelled him to become a teacher, he relinquished his growing practice to accept the demonstratorship of anatomy in the Medical College of Ohio, at Cincinnati.

His stay at Easton had not been barren in additions to his scientific acquirements. He was constantly at work in a dissecting-room which he built at the foot of his garden. Here, too, he made a series of most careful observations on the rapidity with which articles taken into the stomach are excreted by the kidneys; and investigated the temperature of the venous blood, which he found as an average to be 96 Fahr. Further, he wrote a considerable part of a treatise on descriptive anatomy, in which an English in place of a Latin nomenclature was employed. This work was never finished; the experiments on the blood were published at Cincinnati in the second volume of the Western Medical Gazette.

As a demonstrator in the Medical College of Ohio, which he joined in the autumn of 1833, Dr. Gross was very successful. But he did not long remain in this position; for after the work of two sessions he accepted the Chair of Pathological Anatomy in the Medical Department of the Cincinnati College. He threw himself with even more than his usual ardor into the subject, and the number of specimens he studied and collected was great, and the extent of his reading enormous.

It was the pursuit of Pathological Anatomy, on which he gave the first systematic course delivered in this country, which made him so learned and skilled a surgical diagnostician, and he cherished through life a great devotion to the branch. Nor was his association with it limited to the four years he taught it from the professor's chair. His "Elements of Pathological Anatomy," issued in 1839 in two octavo volumes of more than five hundred pages each, did more to attract attention to the subject than anything that had ever been done in this country. The book, illustrated profusely with woodcuts and with several colored engravings, reached three editions. It is a mine of learning, and its extended references make it valuable to this day.

Its merits have been fully recognized abroad; and on no occasion more flatteringly than when the great pathologist, Virchow, at a dinner given to Dr. Gross at Berlin in 1863, complimented him publicly on being the author, and, pointing to the volume which he laid upon the table, gracefully acknowledged the pleasure and instruction with which he had often consulted it. As another acknowledgment of its merits, we find that soon after the publication of the second edition the Imperial Royal Society of Vienna made Dr. Gross an honorary member.

Dr. Gross remained six years in Cincinnati, popular as a teacher, and gradually acquiring a large general practice; but with a stronger and stronger predilection for surgery. It was this chiefly which led him to accept the Professorship of Surgery in the University of Louisville; and with the removal to Louisville in 1840 Dr. Gross' national reputation may be said to begin. Patients flocked in on him from all sides. He soon became the leading surgeon of the Southwest, being often called away long distances into the interior of Kentucky and adjacent States. He lived in a large house in a very hospitable manner, and with a young family around him the house was gay and pleasant, and a centre for men and women of mark.

But neither the claims of practice, nor the demands of social life, quenched his thirst for work. He published, besides many papers in the Western Journal of Medicine and Surgery, a most valuable monograph on the "Nature and Treatment of Wounds of the Intestines," which contained many original experiments and observations. He printed full biographies of Daniel Drake and of Ephraim McDowell—the surgeon who had the boldness to be the first to perform ovariotomy, and through whose boldness, it has been computed, thousands of years have been added to human life.

He wrote a lengthy report on the "Results of Surgical Operations in Malignant Disease," published a treatise on "Diseases of the Urinary Organs," which soon became an acknowledged authority, and has passed through several editions; wrote a work on "Foreign Bodies in the Air Passages," from which all subsequent authors have largely copied their facts, and of which the distinguished laryngologist, Morrell Mackenzie, has declared that it is doubtful whether it ever will be improved upon.

Part of all the enormous labors necessary to complete these and other literary undertakings was performed in New York, where Dr. Gross passed the winter of 1850-51, occupying the Chair of Surgery in the University of New York, which had been rendered vacant by the retirement of the then most famous operative surgeon of this country, Valentine Mott. But, however pleasant he found the social life of the great city, he deemed it best for his own interests not to tarry there, and he returned to Louisville; his late colleagues received him with open arms, and his successor, Dr. Eve, with generous abnegation, retired to let him renew his teachings from his old chair. It seemed that nothing would again take Dr. Gross away from Louisville, where he became a very prominent citizen, in whose reputation all took pride.

But in the spring of 1856 came the offer which he had not the heart to resist; the call from his Alma Mater to fill the Chair of Surgery, vacated by the most popular professor of the branch in this country; the idol of the largest classes then assembling in any medical school in America. To succeed Thomas D. Mutter was a trial to any one. But Dr. Gross, conscious of his powers as a teacher, in the prime of life and of vigor, ambitious to connect his name forever with that of the College where he had been educated and which a band of eminent men had made so flourishing, accepted the task without misgivings, and the result was unmixed success for himself and great benefit to the Institution.

Many were the remonstrances against his leaving the home of his adoption, and he did so, he tells us himself in his inaugural address, against the inclinations and wishes of his family. Moreover, he was very loth to sever his connection with the University of Louisville "for sixteen years the pride and solace of my professional life." And it was the simple truth when he stated that in making the change and coming to Philadelphia, he, the most noted surgeon of the Southwest, had left behind him an empire of Surgery.

His inaugural address was very favorable received. His impressive voice, his splendid intellectual appearance, the earnestness and force of his words, the latent power which all his utterances and actions showed, carried away his audience; and when in solemn tones he spoke these words of his peroration "Whatever of life, and of health, and of strength, remains to me, I hereby, in the presence of Almighty God and of this large assemblage, dedicate to the cause of my Alma Mater, to the interests of Medical Science, and to the good of my fellow-creatures," it was felt that a man of great strength and earnest endeavor had come among us.

Never were thoughts more faithfully put into action. Dr. Gross was indefatigable, and became a celebrated teacher, deeply devoted to the school, the reputation of which he enhanced greatly. Indeed, it may be said, without injustice to any one, that for years he was the most commanding figure and the most popular teacher in it. Nor is it enough to judge him only by those around him or who held similar chairs in other institutions. It is not the recollection of many acts of encouraging kindness from an older to a younger man; it is not the pride of a colleague in the great reputation of one to whom all looked up,—which makes the writer of these lines say that in his professional life Samuel D. Gross takes rank with the very few of the most renowned teachers of his day.

To assign him his proper position he must be named with the Hyrtls, the Trousseaus, the Pagets. Less finished in eloquence he may have been, but in perspicuity and impressiveness and in influence on his hearers he was not one whit behind. Seeing him standing in his lecture room, you saw the man at his best. The learning, the method of his discourse, its clearness and fullness were not more admirable than the force and directness of the words which, uttered in his deep and agreeable voice, sank into the minds of his youthful audience. Years afterwards men whose hair was turning gray would cite the strong words of the lesson the great teacher had made part of the guiding thought of their daily lives.

His didactic lectures were probably his best, though his clinical discourses were also models of perspicuity. He was least happy in his addresses, delivered as introductories or valedictories, or on special occasions. During his long and busy life he wrote many of them, some of considerable historical value, such as the Life of Mott, of John Hunter, a discourse on Ambrose Paré, an oration in honor of Ephraim McDowell.

As these discourses were always written out, he read them from manuscript. But he was not a good reader, and no one to hear him would suppose that it was the same man who, great professor that he certainly was, had, when speaking without notes to his class, their upflagging, devoted attention. Strange to say, too, for one who wrote so well, the addresses show faults which appear nowhere else. They do not possess the art of leaving things unsaid, hence there at times repetitions in them, marring their general efficiency. They have force—for it was impossible for this strong man to do anything that has not force—but they lack literary perspective.

Nothing of the kind, however, appears in his scientific writings. On the contrary, they are as concise, as vivid as it is possible to be. Nothing but strong thoughts, nothing but clear words. And Dr. Gross acquired this excellent style to such perfection that he wrote pages without a single correction. A most critical proof-reader once informed the writer, that of all the authors he had ever known, Dr. Gross altered least, his proof was the cleanest, there was scarcely a correction to be made or suggested.

His literary pursuits were unremitting during his residence in Philadelphia. Memoirs, reviews, essays on surgical subjects appeared in rapid succession; no sooner was one done than another was under way. In conjunction with Dr. T. G. Richardson, he was editor of a flourishing journal, the North American Medical Chirurgical Review. He was also editor of, as well as chief contributor to a volume bearing the title of "Lives of Eminent American Physicians and Surgeons of the Nineteenth Century." And in 1876, as a contribution to the literature of the Centennial year, appeared a lengthy and extraordinary learned history of American Surgery from 1776 to 1876.

As an instance of the rapid manner in which, if necessary, he could work, may be mentioned, that at the outbreak of the Civil War, he composed a pocket manual of Military Surgery in nine days, which was largely used by the young surgeons in the service of the United States, was soon republished in Richmond and equally employed by the surgeons of the Southern armies. A Japanese translation of this little work appeared in 1874, and is still in use among the military surgeons of this enterprising nation.

But the great work he competed in Philadelphia, one by which his name will be long remembered, is his "System of Surgery," a work of which the first edition was published in two very large, profusely illustrated octavo volumes in 1859, and which in 1882 reached its sixth edition. The labor on it, and on the successive editions which brought it up to its present perfection, was enormous. Rising early, working late, writing with an assiduity that only a man of his wonderful physique could have kept up, he generally gave from five to eight hours a day to the cherished project, no matter what the interruptions or whatever else he had to do. Often, too, he would think out, while driving about town on his professional visits, the subject he was engaged on, and commit these thoughts to paper on his return home, before he took rest or food.

The treatise on Surgery has become everywhere a standard authority. "His work is cosmopolitan, the surgery of the world being fully represented in it," says the Dublin Journal of Medical Science. "Long the standard work on the subject for students and practitioners," is the verdict of the London Lancet of May of this year, on the twenty-three hundred and eighty-two pages of the last edition. A Dutch translation was issued in 1863.

Dr. Gross always took the keenest interest in every question relating to his own profession and in its honor and advancement. He was a very constant visitor at Medical Societies in various parts of the United States and in Great Britain. He was probably known personally to more physicians and men of science than any other man in the United States, and wherever he went he had many followers and admirers. Most of the prominent surgeons of England were his personal friends.

His interest in Medical Societies never flagged, and late in life he became the founder of two very flourishing ones, of the Academy of Surgery of Philadelphia and of the American Surgical Association. He served as president of both. In 1868 we find him as President of the American Medical Association at its meeting in Washington; and in 1876 as the President of an International Medical Congress in session at Philadelphia.

He was a member of most of the noted medical societies of this country, of the Academy of Natural Sciences, and of this Society. He was also a member of many learned societies abroad; among them, of the Royal Medical Chirurgical Society of London, the Clinical Society of London, the Imperial Medical Society of Vienna, the Medical Society of Christiana, the Royal Society of Public Medicine of Belgium. But his highest foreign honors were conferred upon him by the three great English Universities. D.C.L. of Oxford, in 1872, at the one thousandth commemoration of the University; LL.D. of Cambridge in 1880, in the same list with Brown-Sequard, with Donders, with Joseph Lister; LL.D. of Edinburgh in absentia, a compliment the more marked since it was only shared with Tennyson and a few others of great distinction,—the renowned American Surgeon carried honors which few of his countrymen have ever borne together.

His welcome at Oxford on Commemoration Day was very enthusiastic. His commanding appearance made him conspicuous even among the distinguished men who surrounded him, and a lady who was present told the writer that she felt a glow of patriotic pride in witnessing his warm reception and hearing the flattering remarks his splendid bearing elicited. At Cambridge the Public Orator addressed him as "Patriae nostrae ad portus nuper advectus est vir venerabilis quem inter fratres nostros Transatlanticos scientiae Chirurgicae quasi alterum Nestorem nominare ausim." Of American colleges, to their shame be it spoken, only two, Jefferson College in 1861 and the University of Pennsylvania in 1884, bestowed on him any honorary degree in recognition of his great literary and scientific merit.

In March, 1882, Dr. Gross found that his physical strength was scarcely adequate to the arduous labors of his chair, and, while mentally as fit as ever, he resigned his cherished Professorship of Surgery. The trustees at once elected him Emeritus Professor, and it was a great gratification to him to find that, in dividing the chair into two, they selected his son, Dr. Samuel W. Gross, to fill one part of it.

The remaining years of Dr. Gross's life were passed in pleasant retirement, but not idly. He had for years in Philadelphia been busy as a consulting Surgeon and in a large office practice, and to a certain amount of this he attended to the last, his great reputation bringing him still many a patient from a distance. He also wrote diligently on an autobiography, published a paper "On the value of early operations in Morbid Growths;" another "On the best means of Training Nurses for the Rural Districts," a subject in which he was much interested; and composed two essays, one of them, on "Wounds of the Intestines," but a few weeks before his death.

His hospitality, his genial manners were the same as ever; nay, advancing years softened the whole man, and made him more benign and more and more beloved. He was delightful in his own home, always surrounded by friends, adored by his family. The best of fathers, he had the constant companionship and care of the most devoted of children.

In the autumn of 1883 he showed symptoms of a weak heart; his feet were swollen, partly from dropsy, partly from rheumatic gout, and he had a long attack of bronchial catarrh. But he improved and held his own fairly well, notwithstanding signs that his digestive functions were failing, until after a severe cold in March, these began to give way entirely, and he died of exhaustion, May the 6th, after a long and most trying illness, which he all along regarded as his last. The deepest sympathy and affection were everywhere expressed for him. Telegrams and letters came daily, inquiring after him; old pupils, busy men, traveled hundreds of miles to grasp him once more by the hand. To very many his death was a deep personal sorrow.

An autopsy, made at his own request, showed that the stomach and heart were degenerating. He had lived out the life of possible strength; to have lived longer would have been to enter upon a life of suffering. His death saved him from protracted inaction and pain, from what Heine, in his own case, has pathetically bewailed as the "mattress grave." By special directions in Dr. Gross's will the body was cremated, and the ashes have been placed beside the coffin of his wife in Woodlands Cemetery.

Such is a sketch of the life of this prodigious worker. An original contributor to the science for which he had a fondness; a widely known practical surgeon; an admirable, most learned writer; a great teacher exerting an influence which will long survive him,—Dr. Gross occupied the foremost rank in the medical profession. It was evident from his student days that he was to be a man of rare distinction:

> "Mens ardus semper
> A puero, tenerisque etiam fulgebat in annis
> Fortunae majoris honos."

He, certainly, was of the men whose high fortune throws its shadows before from the earliest years. The youth showed what the mature man was; the old man was but the youth with the promise fulfilled, and with honors gracefully worn that no one ever doubted would be attained.

A part of his extraordinary fame is due to the circumstances under which he worked. He was the first writer on this continent who, with anything like gift of expression, brought together and elaborated the truths of surgical science, and partly this, but chiefly the excellence of his labors, extended his reputation in all directions beyond his own country. In acquiring fame for himself, he added to her fame. Conspicuous in many ways, Samuel Dent Gross stands forth a marked personality among the eminent men of our or of any generation.

EDITORS' NOTE

Samuel D. Gross was as great a surgeon as the US produced in the 19th century. His colleagues referred to him as the "Emperor of American Surgery." Not surprisingly the memoir written by his disciple Dr. DeCosta omits an important blemish on Gross' otherwise stellar career—his stubborn and highly influential opposition to antisepsis. Also not mentioned in the memoir is the reason that Dr. Gross' fame has endured or even increased in the 21st Century, his depiction as the surgeon in Thomas Eakins Gross Clinic, considered by some art critics to be America's best painting. Ten years before the time of the painting Joseph Lister had introduced antiseptic technique and it had already been widely accepted in Europe, preventing many deaths from postoperative infection.

In the painting Gross' disregard of antisepsis is obvious from his unsterile garb, instruments and hands. WW Keen (APS 1884, see pp. 126) recalled that Gross sometimes paused during operations to sharpen his knife on the sole of his boot. A few young American surgeons including Keen were stimulated to practice antisepsis by their attendance of Lister's demonstration of his techniques during his visit to Philadelphia in 1876. But for another 10 years many surgical patients in the U.S. lost their lives from infection because American surgeons followed Samuel Gross' advice and refused to adopt antiseptic techniques.

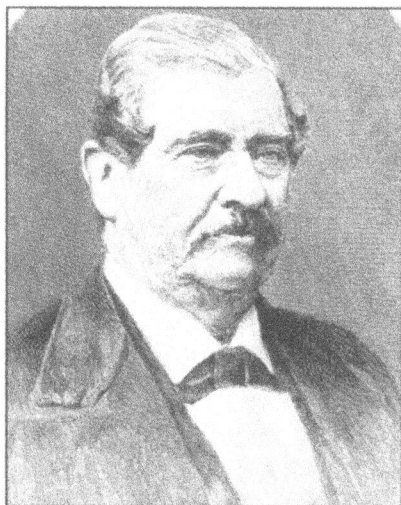

ROBERT E. ROGERS

1813–1884 (APS 1855)

Memoir by W. S. W. Ruschenberger

After Dr. Robert E. Rogers died in 1884, Dr. W.S.W. Ruschenberger was assigned the obituary. He fulfilled this obligation with a 33 page description of the lives and accomplishments of Dr. Rogers, his three brothers, and their Irish immigrant father, Patrick Kerr Rogers. An additional nine pages listed the publications of all five men. The 42 page document began as follows:

The life of Dr. Robert E. Rogers was interwoven in many ways with the lives of his three brothers. All were able university professors. They labored jointly as well as separately to increase and diffuse knowledge. On this account they were more or less distinguished. All were members of the American Philosophical Society. All are dead. No obituary minute of either has been recorded in its archives. Therefore it seems proper to group together sketches of the four brothers in such manner as may give to each, if possible, his characteristic features.

Each followed his routine course; but often they engaged jointly in one investigation, so that the public sometimes confounded their labors and gave credit to one which truly belonged to another. Their works were frequently mentioned at home and abroad as of "the brothers Rogers," and always in respectful and kindly terms. Mistakes of the sort never disturbed the perfect harmony that always existed between them, as they might have done had the brothers been rivals or competitors for reputation. Their days of boyhood were passed together in delightful companionship with their father, whom they regarded with profound respect. Their tastes and pursuits were similar. Their home-training taught them to love one another, so they went through life practicing, unconsciously, no doubt,

---

Material in Bold Italic was added by co-editor Thomas E. Starzl

89

the affectionate ways which they had inherited and learned from their mother, a sensible woman of a gentle and loving nature.

Most of the seven ensuing pages of Dr. Ruschenberger's obituary(ies) is devoted to the life and career of the father, Patrick Kerr Rogers (not an APS member), with the following justification:

This sketch of his *[Patrick's]* trying career is presented because the profound, affectionate respect with which the sons always regarded their father, suggests that this commemoration would be unsatisfactory to them in their graves if he were not associated in it. Besides, he seems to have been the mental type of his sons to a considerable degree, though they were indebted to their mother largely for their moral constitution.

The second and third sons (William Barton and Henry Darwin) became famous geologists, scientists, and educators. For example, William founded the Massachusetts Institute of Technology (MIT) and Henry was appointed Regius Professor of Natural History-Geology at Glasgow University and Keeper of the Huntarian museum. Patrick Kerr Rogers (the father) and his first and last sons (James Blythe and Robert Empie Rogers) obtained medical degrees, but did little practice. Instead, they became basic science investigators and educators, primarily in the field of biochemistry. The following excerpts from Dr. Ruschenberger's 42 page "sketch" are primarily concerned with the career of Dr. Robert Empie Rogers, the last born son and decreed focus of the obituary.

Robert Empie Rogers, the sixth child and fourth son of his parents, was born in Baltimore, March 29, 1813. He assumed the name of Empie while a youth as a lasting token of his grateful appreciation of parental care bestowed upon him at the College of William and Mary after the death of his mother, in 1820, when he was only seven years old, by the Rev. Adam P. Empie, D.D., and his wife.

His early education was directed by his father. After his death, 1828, it was managed by his brothers James and William. The intention was that he should be a civil engineer. *His resistance to this plan is expressed in* "...a letter dated...May 6, 1833...to his brother William, at Williamsburg, Va." *in which he reveals his desire to have charge of a school. He states that* "...at no time could I learn so fast as when teaching, for then I should be making practical application of what I would be myself acquiring, and while occupied I would have also a portion of time altogether apart to myself to devote in my own way to my own improvement.... . I was doubtful whether it would be prudent to occupy myself with mathematics until I could be under your direction. I will therefore refrain from the present and continue with botany, geology and mineralogy."

The project of becoming a civil engineer was abandoned. Probably in the autumn of 1833 he determined to study medicine. He became a pupil of Dr. Robert Hare, Professor of Chemistry, and worked zealously in his laboratory till the close of his undergraduate course. He duly submitted a thesis, entitled "Experiments on the blood, together with some new facts in regard to animal and vegetable structures, illustrative of many of the most important phenomena of organic life," etc., and graduated from the Medical Department of the University of Pennsylvania, March, 1836 This thesis, illustrated by many wood cuts, was published in the American Journal of the Medical Sciences. The practice of medicine was not to his taste. He devoted himself to chemistry. From 1836 to 1842 he was the chemist of the first Geological Survey of Pennsylvania, of which his brother Henry was the chief. Near the close of his thirtieth year he married, March 13, 1843, Miss Fanny Montgomery, a daughter of Mr. Joseph S. Lewis, a gentleman who was prominent among those who established the city's water-works at Fairmount.

During this period of his life, Dr. Rogers apparently was physically fit as illustrated by the following anecdote of Dr. Ruschenberger. One Sunday, at Long Branch, years ago, a gentleman who was bathing got beyond his depth and was borne seaward by the undertow. Two young men who were bathing at the same time saw his danger and hastened to his assistance; but when they reached him they were able to do little more than care for themselves. They could only now and then give him a little support and encourage him to continue his exertions to save himself.

Dr. Rogers saw their peril from the hotel and instantly started for the beach, undressing and throwing, his clothes, containing his watch, money, etc., on the ground as he ran, and reached it just in time to jump on board of a boat putting off to the rescue. The boat had proceeded only a short distance when it was swamped. Dr. Rogers seized an oar, swam to the drowning persons, gave it to them and urged them to sustain themselves till aid should arrive. The drifting boat was flung against one of the gentlemen and the oar was wrenched from him. Seeing this, Dr. Rogers placed himself in a manner under him, and thus bearing him up, brought him, as well as those holding fast to the oar, safely ashore. And this was the third time he had heroically saved persons from drowning.

He became a member of the Academy of Natural Sciences, of Philadelphia, February, 1837. During nearly a half century he evinced interest in the pursuits of the Society. At irregular intervals he was frequently present at its stated meetings of several successive years, participated in discussions, delivered lectures to promote its interest and contributed to its funds.

Dr. Rogers was elected a member of the Franklin Institute of the State of Pennsylvania, April 18, 1838. In the session 1841–42, on invitation, he had completed the course of chemical instruction at the University of Virginia which had been interrupted by sickness of the professor, Dr. John P. Emmet, from which he did not recover. Dr. Rogers was elected in his place, Professor of General and Applied Chemistry and Materia Medica, in March, 1842, and discharged the duties of the office in Virginia satisfactorily to all concerned during ten years. He resigned from the Franklin Institute on May 18, 1845 *[but was]* again elected November 18, 1852 on returning to Philadelphia after the *[10 year]* absence; became a "life member" in 1855, and one of the Board of Managers in 1857. He was one of the vice-presidents during seventeen years, from January, 1858.

In January, 1875, he was elected President *of the Institute.* He declined reelection January, 1879, and was again returned to the Board of Managers...*In a footnote, the unanimous reaction of the Institute members was:* "Whereas, Our highly esteemed presiding officer, Dr. R.E. Rogers, having declined a re-election to the office he has so acceptably filled for the past four years, it is therefore, Resolved, That in parting with Dr. Rogers we desire to place on record our high appreciation of the courteous and impartial manner with which he has presided over our deliberations, as well as our appreciation of the valuable time and talents he has devoted to the service of this Institute, and we indulge the hope that In future as In the past, it may have the benefit of his extensive research and great experience."

He was prominently active in the work of the Institute, delivered courses of lectures on chemistry before its classes, assisted in the management of its public exhibitions, served on several of its standing and on many of its special committees, the most notable of which was one on tests of the efficiency of dynamo-electric machines, and another on the dangers of electric lighting. At the celebration of the semi-centennial anniversary of the foundation of the society, February 5, 1874, in the Musical Fund Hall, he delivered an eloquent address, narrating in a general way a history of scientific discoveries and their practical applications in the half century, and indicating how the work carried on during that period by the Institute had contributed to the progress of science and the diffusion of knowledge.

Robert Rogers' role at the University of Pennsylvania was long and distinguished, particularly after returning from his decade stint at the University of Virginia. He was elected Professor of Chemistry in the University of Pennsylvania, August, 1852, in place of his brother James *(who died that year)* and was made Dean of the Medical Faculty in 1856…The American edition of Lehmann's great work, Physiological Chemistry, was edited by him and published by Blanchard & Lea, October, 1855…He was chosen a member of the American Philosophical Society July 30, 1855 *(age 42)*, and elected one of its Council January 7, 1859. He was frequently present at the meetings of the Society, often took part in discussions, and served on several committees.

While the war of rebellion was in progress Dr. Rogers was appointed an Acting Assistant-Surgeon in the army, July 8, 1862, for duty at the West Philadelphia Military Hospital, and served till June 18, 1863. At his suggestion and under his supervision, a steam mangle was set up in West Philadelphia—Chestnut Street, east of Thirty-first Street to accelerate the laundry work of the great hospital. The day the machine was ready to be set to work, January 10, 1863, he was present to see it started. It is related that while benevolently showing a woman who was to feed it the dangers to which the work exposed her, his own right hand was caught and crushed betwixt the very hot [1800° F] revolving iron cylinders. With characteristic alertness he reached out his left hand and instantly threw the leather band off from the revolving drum which gave motion to the machine, and stopped it. Then, in lifting the heavy cylinder [800] pounds for his release, it slipped from the end of a crowbar in the hands of a workman and fell back upon the hand, thus aggravating the injury already inflicted.

In his suffering he was considerate of another. He conjectured that his wife might be too profoundly shocked, should he appear before her with the hurt hand concealed in bloody wraps, immediately after the sound of rattling wheels in their quiet street had ceased in front of the house. To convey to her an impression that his injury was less than it really was, he gallantly alighted from the carriage in which he was at the street corner nearest his residence and walked home.

His colleague in the University, Dr. Henry H. Smith, Professor of Surgery, amputated the injured extremity above the wrist at night, January 24. The result of the operation was entirely satisfactory. For some time he wore an artificial hand, admirably made for him by C. W. Kolbe, a well-known cutler of the city.

One day, very soon after the stump had healed, as Professor Smith was about to begin his lecture, Dr. Rogers entered the arena and begged leave to interrupt him for a moment. Then, resting his left hand upon the Professor's shoulder, he addressed the assembled class in his eloquent way, and expressed his grateful sense of obligation to the eminent skill and kind attention of their Professor of Surgery. His speech was received with rounds of tremendous applause. The scene is not likely to be forgotten by any who was present.

Almost ambidextrous prior to the accident, he speedily learned to write with his left hand and to use the right arm, beneath the shoulder, in prehension with notable skill in his experiments while lecturing. Soon after the loss of his hand a greater sorrow came to him. His happy married life of twenty years was ended. His wife died February 21, 1863. Miss Delia Saunders became his second wife, April 30, 1866.

Portending today's infiltration of basic science into life quotidian, Dr. Roger's advice was sought under diverse circumstances. In 1858, he reported one of the first applications of chemistry to forensic criminology to the College of Physicians of Philadelphia. This was … a case of arsenical poisoning in which he appeared in Court as an expert. The victim had been taking, for some time, subnitrate of bismuth by prescription. He found that a remnant of the same contained a small quantity of arsenic, and also that samples of subnitrate of bismuth, obtained from ten druggists' shops, were contaminated in like manner, but not sufficiently to render the quantity ordinarily prescribed dangerous. On this testimony the jury acquitted the accused, although circumstances strongly implied his guilt. Arsenical contamination of the subnitrate of bismuth of the shops had not been previously suspected.

Dr. Rogers' role in industrial affairs derived in part from his remarkable facility in the use of tools of all kinds, and a respectable talent for mechanical contrivance. He was author of many inventions—notable among them the Rogers and Black steam boiler—and of several modifications and improvements of electric apparatus. This ability was early manifested, 1835–36, in his original experiments on osmosis, in which he demonstrated how changes in the blood are produced by respiration.

His presence in the financial world was greatly enhanced by his involvement with coin currency. On May 10, 1872, the Secretary of the Treasury of the United States appointed Drs. H. R. Linderman and Robert E. Rogers a committee to examine the Melter and Refiner's Department of the Mint at Philadelphia, and ascertain the extent and sources of an alleged "waste of silver in excess of the amount tolerated by law." *After about 2 months* of innumerous experiments, the result of it was presented July 25, 1872, in a well-considered and elaborate "Report on the wastage of silver bullion in the Melter and Refiner's Department of the Mint."

This investigation, valuable in itself, was also valuable in its consequences. His experimental trials to apply the principles of chemical science to the improvement of an industrial process of great importance, suggested modifications in the methods of refining the precious metals which were subsequently adopted. *In one federally-mandated application, Dr. Rogers ...*made, in November, 1875, "a careful and laborious investigation" of the consolidated Virginia and California Mine in Nevada, for the purpose of estimating "their probable total yield of gold and silver based upon their present explored extent and the quality of their ores as ascertained by assays." And after due consideration of the chances of over-estimation he placed the production "at not less than $150,000,000," which is one-half of the sum indicated by the assays.

During the same period (1873–74), Dr. Rogers also was asked to troubleshoot a problem at the San Francisco mint. Nitrous acid fames, arising from the nitric acid used in refining silver, were allowed to escape, through the chimney, into the open air, sometimes seriously annoying neighbors. To correct the evil, Dr. Rogers had constructed in the attic of the building a furnace for burning coke, into which the fumes were conveyed and burned. Instead of extinguishing the fuel these fumes promote its combustion, which is an interesting chemical fact. *Dr. Rogers' solutions* which included the sulphuric acid process ... were adopted May 3, 1875. They included the erection of additional buildings.

Dr. Rogers arrived at San Francisco May 19. The actual work of construction and equipment of the refinery was begun May 24, and finished July 26, and placed in charge of the Superintendent, in working order, August 25, 1875. During the progress of the work, *and at Dr. Rogers' suggestion,* an artesian well was sunk within the hollow square of the Mint which supplies 100,000 gallons of excellent water daily for all the uses of the establishment.

In reference to this enterprise, the Director of the Mint, in his annual report, November 20, 1875, says: "The arranging of the plan of the refinery and its equipment was entrusted to Robert E. Rogers, Professor of Chemistry in the University of Pennsylvania, whose eminent qualifications as a chemist and metallurgist, rendered him peculiarly qualified for this service, and who performed the duty assigned him in an entirely satisfactory manner. The refinery has been in successful operation since the 26th day of August last, and with much advantage to the public interests."

Besides doing the work just mentioned, Dr. Rogers served as a member of the Annual Assay Commission every year from 1874 to 1879, both years included. From June, 1872, till his death, he was one of the chemists, employed by the Gas Trust of Philadelphia, to make analyses and daily photometrical tests of the gas. He was succeeded in the office by his assistant, Dr. George M. Ward.

Dr. Roger's role as chemist in The Pennsylvania geologic survey of 1836-42 (headed by his brother, Henry) uniquely qualified him to advise coal companies and others seeking mineral riches. The results were not always fruitful. Under an attraction of speculative chances in petroleum, which at the time shrewd men believed to be excellent, many friends, relying upon his scientific judgment in the premises, were induced to join Dr. Rogers in organizing the Humboldt Oil Company, February 17, 1864. They contributed a quarter of a million of dollars. Land supposed to be richly stored with oil was purchased, wells were sunk and work carried on for some time without profit. The assets of the company were publicly sold, February 4, 1873, for a sum not more than sufficient to return the stockholders one cent a share. Dr. Rogers owned one-fifth of all the shares, and lost more than any one who had stock in the unhappy enterprise he had prompted.

Collapse of the Humboldt Oil Company in 1873 coincided with the beginning of another chink in Dr. Rogers' previously seamless public image. Very soon after the University of Pennsylvania was transferred to the buildings which it now occupies in West Philadelphia, it was suggested that the scheme of medical teaching which had been long followed ought to be improved. During the evolution of the plan adopted and the transition from the old to the new ways, personal discussions of the subject were frequent and often warm. The Board of Trustees, it was supposed, did not rightly appreciate the injury which the proposed changes might work to its medical faculty. The professors were ready for and in favor of such reform as would make the diploma significant of qualifications higher than obtainable in any other medical school; but they were not prepared to sacrifice their pecuniary interests...

Rivalry and competition of the many medical schools are strong, each striving to attract as many students as possible, because, as a rule, the emolument of the professors is contingent upon the number; and large classes, in common estimation, vouch for the excellence of the school as well as of the qualification of its graduates. The circumstances of medical teaching suggested that to immediately prolong the course of study, thus augmenting the expenses of the student and increase the requirements of graduation to what they should be, must be instantly followed by great reduction of the classes, and consequently of the remuneration of the professors. The aspect of affairs was to them unpromising. Discontent was prevalent.

While matters were still in an uncertain state, Dr. Rogers, without application, was elected, May 2, 1877, Professor of Medical Chemistry and Toxicology in the Jefferson Medical College, a chair just vacated by resignation. He accepted the office and resigned his position in the University *(chemistry Chair and Dean)*, which he had held during a quarter of a century. The transfer added to his emolument without increase of labor and relieved his anxiety.

The Trustees managed affairs wisely. They established the excellent scheme of medical education now in operation, which, followed thoroughly by the student, places him beyond the necessity of seeking further instruction after graduation in post-graduate courses, which many to whom diplomas may have been prematurely granted consider essential to properly qualify them for general practice. Discontent has disappeared. The professors receive annual salaries in place of fees from students. The prosperity of the Medical Department of the University seems to be assured.

The reception of Dr. Rogers into the Jefferson Medical College was cordially manifested at his lecture introductory to the course of 1877–78. It was estimated that not less than 1200 physicians, students and others were crowded into the hall. At the conclusion of the lecture a silver vase was presented to him as a token of the respect felt for him by the great class of medical students. In addition to his own work in the college he completed the course of instruction on Materia Medica in the session of 1878, left unfinished by the professor of that branch, Dr. John B. Biddle, who died January 19, 1879. The degree of Doctor of Laws, LL.D., was conferred upon him June, 1883, by Dickinson College, Carlisle, PA.

His second wife died January 9, 1883. This loss made a profound impression. Abated energy and impaired health followed. He resigned his office, July, 1884, and was elected emeritus professor. He died September 6, 1884, in his seventy-second year.

EDITORS' NOTE

In 1874 the University of Pennsylvania moved the locus of its patient based teaching from Pennsylvania Hospital, a private independent institution in Center City to a newly constructed hospital in West Philadelphia. It was the Nation's first University owned and controlled hospital. This triggered a dispute that culminated in the defection to Jefferson by the Medical Schools' long term dean, Robert Rogers.

For patient based teaching of medical students in the new hospital the University's trustees had appointed a staff, which they termed "clinical professors." Unlike the established professors of the school, they did not at first have university appointments and thus were not allowed to give the student lectures or sign diplomas. The entrenched university professors were opposed to granting the clinical professors these and other rights that would make the newcomers' status equal to their own. One reason was that the university professors were paid directly for their lectures by the students. This revenue stream would be threatened by upgraded clinical professors. At the same time, there was a proposal under discussion to increase the medical school from two to three years. The university professors also resisted this, predicting that it would decrease the number of students attending Penn, further diminishing their income.

Dr. Rogers as dean sided with his university faculty in an effort to maintain the status quo. After bitter discussions and failed compromises the trustees elected to give the hospital's clinical professors full university appointments, including privileges to lecture and to sign diplomas. In addition student fees for lectures were no longer to be paid to the professors but instead to the school which would then provide salaries to its faculty. Having lost the war, Dr. Rogers resigned and moved to Jefferson.

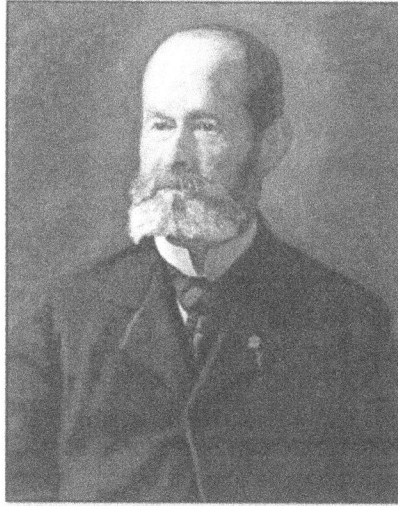

DANIEL GARRISON BRINTON

1837–1899 (APS 1869)

Memoir by Albert H. Smyth

We have met to do honor to an illustrious scholar, in whose death we mourn the loss of one who has redeemed American scholarship from any taint of narrowness or charge of incompletion.

It is easy for us to lift our hearts in praise of him, but it is difficult to deal justly and adequately, in the brief time allowed to me, with one who touched life on so many sides, and who won high distinction and conferred signal benefits in so many and diverse fields. He would have been the first to reprove extravagant eulogy, for in his modesty he took little credit to himself for achievements that were of worldwide importance and acceptance. He knew the immensity of the untraveled world before him, and, single-hearted in the pursuit of truth, he counted not himself to have attained, but to be still patiently working toward that far-off goal of all intellectual endeavor.

Everywhere, at seats of learning, in erudite societies, and among distinguished scholars—the name of Daniel Garrison Brinton is known and honored. American scholarship in him commanded respect and won the recognition of the world. If at home his great talents were not always appreciated to the height, and he was not invested with that authority and preeminence which justly belonged to him, it is but another distinguished illustration of the truth of Cardinal Newman's high saying, that "the saints live in sackcloth, and are buried in silk and purple."

In his own particular field of American ethnology he was without a peer, but his intellectual interests were unusually broad, and in widely different spheres of science and literature he commanded respectful attention. Those who knew him were impressed by his encyclopaedic knowledge and they admired the symmetry of his culture. He wrought, not from curiosity or vain ambition, but with a controlling sincerity, at many widely different studies. He was steeped in the classics, a diligent reader of many modern literatures, a careful student of the history of art, well trained in the physical sciences, and a bold speculator in philosophy.

The most notable fact about him was his many-sidedness. He had the liveliest interest in all scientific progress. He was in continual fence with men in every sphere of activity, for he never met a man from whom he did not seek to learn something. And his vision was clearer and keener in particulars because of his many-sidedness. It was Emerson who said that "a man is like a bit of Labrador spar which has no lustre as you turn it in your hand until you come to a particular angle, then it shows deep and beautiful colors," but in Dr. Brinton's life each facet and angle had its lustre.

Darwin regretted that his unremitted attention to science had destroyed his power of appreciating poetry and the drama. No such atrophy was possible in the varied intellectual experience of Dr. Brinton. He "dwelt enlarged in alien modes of thought." He took his recreation often in the less-known fields of literature, and one of his chief joys was the discovery of a new author. He introduced a small coterie with keen enthusiasm to the poems of Clarence Mangan. And he was himself the author of an historical drama in blank verse.

When he died—July 31, 1899—his life-work was practically done. He left no great work unfinished, though to the last he was fertile with new ideas and busy with new projects. He lived the life of a retired scholar, but it was not a life of apathetic monotony. In the truest sense he lived in the full stream of the world. He kept pace with the march of mind. The great questions of religion, politics, society and science were of vital importance to him. "Humani nihil a me alienum puto," he might have well said. To these high things he was neither indifferent nor silent. This patient student of difficult American lore did much to connect learning with the living forces of society. In the press and on the lecture platform he served his generation with the same habitual reference to truth that characterized his labors in that obscure mine from which he brought the rich materials of his great works upon the ethnology of the American race.

Daniel Garrison Brinton was a native of Pennsylvania, born at Thornbury, in Chester county, May 13, 1837. He was descended from English Quakers, who came to the colony of Pennsylvania in 1684. William Brinton, the first to come to America, was from Nether Gournall, on the borders of Salop, in which county the first of the name known to history, Robertus de Brinton, was given the manor of Longford by Henry I, which was held by his descendants for several centuries.

Upon the hereditary farm in Chester county was a "village site" of some ancient encampment of the Delaware Indians. Brinton's boyish curiosity was excited by the curious fragments of Indian pottery which the ploughshare turned out; and with the collections which he made of flint arrowheads and stone axes probably began his interest in the studies which he was destined so mightily to advance. The books which chiefly influenced him while yet a child, and which with a child's eagerness he read and read again, were McClintock's *Antiquarian Researches* and Humboldt's *Cosmos*. They formed his taste and shaped his ambition.

He was prepared for college by Rev. William E. Moore, of West Chester, and he entered Yale College, September 13, 1854. Those who knew him then remember his fondness for recondite learning, and his keen delight in old forgotten folios. He won the second prize for English composition the first term, and the first prize in the second term. In 1857 he became editor of the Yale literary magazine. From 1858, when he took his B.A. at Yale, until 1860 he studied in the Jefferson Medical College. For a year he traveled in Europe, studying in Paris and Heidelberg, and returned to practise medicine at West Chester.

In August, 1862, he entered the army as acting assistant surgeon, and, after passing a second examination in November, 1862, received a commission as surgeon U. S. Volunteers, February 9, 1863. He saw much active service, for he was assigned to duty with the 11th Corps of the Army of the Potomac, as Surgeon-in-Chief of Division, and he was at Chancellorsville, Gettysburg, and other important battles of the war.

After Chickamauga he was sent with the corps to reinforce Rosecrans in East Tennessee, and took part in the battles of Lookout Mountain and Missionary Ridge. In November, 1863, he was made Medical Director of the 11th Corps, and served until April, 1864, when, at his own request, he was transferred to the U.S. Army General Hospital, at Quincy, Ill., and assigned as Surgeon in charge. Here he remained until August 5, 1865, when he was brevetted Lieutenant-Colonel of Volunteers "for meritorious services," and honorably discharged from the army.

In the autumn of 1863 he suffered a sunstroke which compelled his retirement from field duty, and from which he believed he never entirely recovered. He concealed his infirmity with Spartan care, but there was always present with him the apprehension of apoplexy, and that craved cautious living.

He married, September 28, 1865, Miss Sarah Tillson, of Quincy, Ill., and after his marriage he resided in West Chester, and practised medicine until he removed to Philadelphia, and became assistant editor of a weekly publication called The Medical and Surgical Reporter. In 1874 he became editor, and from this time retired from the practice of medicine and devoted himself to editorial work. After twenty years' connection with the Medical and Surgical Reporter he retired in 1887, in order to dedicate himself more completely to the studies which were the passion of his life.

To cite the titles of all his publications would savor of pedantry; and his literary life was so varied and so busy that a mere catalogue of his industry would more than fill the time permitted to this brief address. In the forty years of earnest toil between 1859, when he published his first work, The Floridian Peninsula, and 1899, when he left unfinished his hand-book of "racial psychology," Dr. Brinton wrote twenty-three books and a vast miscellany of pamphlets, monographs and brochures. He contributed forty-eight articles to the Transactions and Proceedings of the American Philosophical Society, and eighty-two papers, of which I have a record, to the Proceedings of other learned bodies and to scientific periodicals.

He printed in the American Historical Magazine studies of "The Mound Builders of the Mississippi Valley" and of "The Shawnees and Their Migrations." In the American Journal of Arts and Sciences he discussed "The Ancient Phonetic Alphabet of Yucatan"; in the American Antiquarian, "The Chief God of the Algonquins in His Character as a Cheat and a Liar." Archaeological articles were furnished by him to the Encyclopaedia Britannica and the Iconographic Encyclopaedia, and many of the articles from his unwearied pen appeared in foreign publications, in the Annales del Museo Nacional, the Revue de Linguistique, and the Compte Rendus of the "Congres International des Americanistes."

It is a wide range of studies that is presented by these multifarious papers. He travels from articles on the "Chontallis and Popolucas" to the "Folk-Lore of the Bones." We turn over his pamphlets and find in quick succession "Notes on the Classical Murmex," "On the Measurement of Thought as Function," on "Left-handedness in North American Aboriginal Art," and "The Etrusco-Libyan Elements in the Song of the Arval Brethren."

In 1882 he began editing and publishing the "Library of American Aboriginal Literature." It is with no inconsiderable solicitude that I venture to speak of that monument of learning, which is one of the most notable scientific enterprises of this country. It is a work of such a kind and such a magnitude that it placed its editor among the first anthropologists of the world, and in pure science ranked him with Whitney and Leidy among the departed, and Furness and Lea among the living. Of this "Library" eight volumes were issued, the first in 1882, the eighth in 1890, and they were designed "to put within reach of scholars authentic materials for the study of the languages and culture of the native races of America."

The volumes appeared in the following order:

No. I. The Chronicles of the Mayas, containing five brief chronicles in the Maya language written shortly after the conquest, and carrying the history of that people back many centuries.

No. II. The Iroquois Book of Rites. Edited by Horatio Hale.

No. III. The Comedy-Ballet of Gueguence. A curious and unique specimen of the native comic dances, with dialogues, called bailes, formerly common in Central America.

No. IV. A Migration Legend of the Creek Indians. Edited by A. S. Gatschet.

No. V. The Lenape and Their Legends. Contains the original text and translation of the 184 symbols of the "Walum Olum," or "Red Score" of the Delaware Indians.

No. VI. The Annals of the Cakchiquels, one of the most important historical documents of the pre-Columbian period.

No. VII. Ancient Nahuatl Poetry, translation and commentary upon twenty-seven songs in the original Nahuatl.

No. VIII. Rig Veda Americanus. Twenty sacred chants of the ancient Mexicans.

I must very briefly characterize Dr. Brinton's other important ethnological and linguistic studies. The American Race, a volume of four hundred pages, was the first attempt at a systematic classification of all the tribes of America, North, Central and South, on the basis of language. It defines seventy-nine linguistic stocks in North America and sixty-one in South America. The number of tribes named and referred to these stocks is nearly 1600. Several of these stocks Dr. Brinton defined for the first time.

In all these difficult and often entirely new explorations into the untraveled region of American languages, he proceeded, not as a mere dialectician, but with a constant reference of special facts to general linguistic theory. He belonged to the non-metaphysical school of philology. That he did not speculate upon language was a self-imposed restraint, for he had a large knowledge of the great work of Whitney, and was well equipped to deal theoretically with dialects and stocks.

However minute the object of his study, it was highly characteristic of him that he never left it without showing its relation to comprehensive general truths. For in addition to his great memory he had an electrical power of combination, which is found only in the greatest scholars, whereby what else were dust from dead men's bones, he brought into the unity of breathing life.

With regard to American languages he was a disciple of Wilhelm von Humboldt and Prof. Steinthal, and he argued that the phenomenon of incorporation in some of its forms is markedly present in the vast majority, if not in all American tongues.

His minutely accurate knowledge of linguistic forms enabled him to spot a forgery with unfailing promptitude. A notable instance was the curious hoax of the Taensa language. The Taensas were a branch of the Natchez, speaking the same tongue. A volume of supposed Taensa writing was printed in the Bibliothèque Linguistique Américaine, but the whole document was conclusively shown by Brinton to be the forgery of some clever young French seminarists. In like manner he demonstrated the fraudulent invention of The Life and Adventures of William Filley, Who was Stolen by the Indians.

His judgment and knowledge were so well understood and respected that he was universally recognized as the final arbiter in all doubtful questions relating to the American race. Upon the authenticity of alleged Indian picture writings or the antiquity of prehistoric bones found in Florida or Alaska he was expected to pass judgment, and his verdict was final.

He contested with unanswerable force the prevalent hypothesis of the Asiatic origin of Mexican and Central American civilization. He rebuked with fine irony the pretensions of those flighty scholars who are now and then off like a rocket for an airy whirl in the clouds. He demanded that the ethnologist should understand and respect the principles of phonetic variation, of systematic derivation, of the historic comparison of languages, of grammatic evolution and morphologic development that, in a word, he should be linked to the shore with towing ropes of science. He concluded his pamphlet On Various Supposed Relations Between the American and Asian Races with these words:

Do any of the numerous languages and innumerable dialects of America present any affinities, judged by the standards of the best modern linguistic schools, which would bring them into genetic relationship with any of the dialects of Asia? I believe I have a right to speak with some authority on this subject, for the American languages have constituted the principal study of my life; and I say unhesitatingly that no such affinities have been shown; and I say this with an abundant acquaintance with such works as The Prehistoric Comparative Philology of Dr. Hyde Clark; with the writings of the Rev. John Campbell, who has discovered the Hittite language in America before we have learned where it was in Asia; with the laborious Comparative Philology of Mr. R. P. Greg; with the Amerikanisch-Asiatische Etymologien of the ardent Americanist Mr. Julius Platzmann; with the proof that the Nahuatl is an Aryan language furnished by the late Director of the National Museum of Mexico, Senor Gumesindo Mendoza; with Varnhagen's array of evidence that the Tupi and Carib are Turanian dialects imported into Brazil from Liberia; with the Abbe Petitot's conviction that the Tinneh of Canada is a Semitic dialect; with Naxera's identification of the Otomi with the Chinese; and with many more such scientific vagaries which, in the auctioneer's phrase, are too tedious to mention.

When I see volumes of this character, many involving prolonged and arduous research on the part of the authors and a corresponding sacrifice of pleasant things in other directions, I am affected by a sense of deep commiseration for able men who expend their efforts in pursuit of such will-o'-the-wisps of science, panting along roads which lead nowhere, inattentive to the guide-posts which alone can direct them to solid ground.

Brinton's studies in the origin and character of the native religions of the Western Continent, which began with The Myths of the New World: A Treatise on the Symbolism and Mythology of the Red Race of America, and were continued in American Hero Myths, found their natural fruition in the important work entitled The Religious Sentiment: A Contribution to the Science and Philosophy of Religions.

The science of religion continued to occupy his thought until in 1897 he published his lectures upon Religions of Primitive Peoples, in some respects his chief contribution to the literature of science. He eloquently interpreted the doctrine of mental unity, arguing for the spontaneous genesis of religion, contending that parallel opinions prevailing among widely separated people did not prove a derivation of ideas. The main thesis of the volume, that the human mind is everywhere in direct contact with the divine, and that therefrom results a spontaneous origination of religious belief, seems to be almost a reminiscence of the Quakerism in which Dr. Brinton was bred.

Brinton was not a sequestered scholar. He delighted to talk with men. He never praised cloistered virtues or sympathized with the ascetic life. In private friendship he was loyal and delightful; in social companionship, easy, polished, good-humored, the ideal of complete gentlemanhood. He was an image of integrity, simplicity and taste, always eager to acknowledge the merits of his fellow-students, always ready to help others at hard parts of the way. His friends loved him, and he never disappointed or repelled. He was tolerant, gentle, self-denying, of most democratic temper—equally at home in the company of scholars, peers or laborers.

His love of social intercourse and his sense of obligation to the great guild of intellect and scholarship brought him into membership in many societies. Twenty-six American societies are represented at this Memorial meeting, and he was a member of at least as many more in France, Italy, Germany, Russia and Spain. He belonged, for example, to the Anthropological Societies of Berlin and Vienna, the Ethnographical Societies of Paris and Florence, the Royal Society of Antiquaries at Copenhagen, and the Royal Academy of History of Madrid. He was medaled by the Société Américaine de France, diplomatized by Yale and the University of Pennsylvania, a Founder of the Reale Società Didascalica Italiana and an Officier de l'Instruction Publique.

He was professor of Ethnology and Archaeology in the Academy of Natural Sciences in Philadelphia, Professor of American Linguistics and Archaeology in the University of Pennsylvania, a President of the Numismatic and Antiquarian Society of Philadelphia, President of the American Association for the Advancement of Science, President of the American Folk-Lore Society, and Vice-President of the International Congress of Américanistes, at Paris.

He became a member of the American Philosophical Society, April 16, 1869. He was elected Curator, January 5, 1877, and continued in office until the close of 1897. He was a Secretary of the Society from January 2, 1880, until the close of 1895. And he was Chairman of the Publication Committee at the time of his death. He was appointed to represent this Society at the following Congresses:

Congrès des Américanistes, at Copenhagen, September, 1884.
Congrès des Américanistes, at Stockholm, September, 1894.
Congrès des Amérianistes, at Havre, 1897.
And he also represented the Society at the memorial meeting
in honor of Dr. G. Brown Goode, 1897.

In conversation and in correspondence he gave freely and generously of his astonishing stores of wide and accurate knowledge. He wrote fluently and talked eloquently, and upon the lecture platform was extremely happy in the art of clear and cogent statement. He worked patiently to improve his style in both written and spoken discourse. Through his successive volumes the attentive reader may observe the constant gain of power and freedom of expression until he is delighted by the grace and mobility of diction in The Pursuit of Happiness and Religions of Primitive Peoples. With like patience and persistence he overcame natural disabilities of speech and gave tone and character to a voice that was unpleasantly marked by the wiry twang of Southern Pennsylvania.

I have already referred to his interest in art and literature. Few men were more familiar than he with the great galleries of Europe, and he had an unusual acquaintance with the poetry of many languages. He was catholic in his tastes. He frequently spoke and read before the Browning Society; he was an ardent admirer of Walt Whitman; and he said that he had often gone to Tennyson for light upon scientific perplexities. His admiration of Walt Whitman and his fondness for the realism of Ibsen and Zola proceeded doubtless from his scientific training. Music was the only art in which he professed no enjoyment. He was fond of quoting Jules Janin: "Music is an expensive noise."

In 1897 he published Maria Candelaria: An Historic Drama from American Aboriginal Life. The scene of the drama is the extreme southeastern State of the Republic of Mexico, and the story is taken from the life of Cancuc, or Maria Candelaria, an Indian girl, a priestess of the Nagualists and the heroine of the revolt of the Tzentals in 1712, whom Dr. Brinton calls "the American Joan of Arc." It was written in blank verse which is smooth and agreeable albeit slightly mechanical.

Brinton knew that the highest art is the art to live. In his Pursuit of Happiness he says, "What nobler compliment could be paid a man than this, which Vittoria Colonna wrote to Michael Angelo, 'You have disposed the labor of your whole life as one single great work of art'?" His sympathies were as many-sided as his knowledge. Social and religious questions which affected individuality and the conduct of life were the subjects of deepest interest and concern to him. "The aim of Science," he said, "is the Real; of Art, the Idea; of Action, Happiness. It is for religion to unite this trinity into a unity in each individual life."

The sentiment of religion was strongly innate in his character. He was naturally reverent, and he always protested against the heedless surrender of legitimate pieties which elevate and consecrate human life. One frequently comes, in his philosophical reflections, upon such a sentence as "We are justified in retaining a reasonable and holy hope that the victory of the grave is not eternal." But his faith never fixed itself to form. He had no sympathy with dogma.

Upon such questions he sometimes spoke before the Ethical Culture Society, and he was always fearless though modest in the presentation of his views, however much they might be at variance with the thought of the time. He stood at all times for individualism, saying "The greatest teachers have not desired disciples, but friends. They have never exerted authority, and when they could not persuade or convince they have sought no proselytes. To them the independence of the individual mind has been of more importance than the dissemination of any article of faith or element of instruction. Spinoza, Herder, Wilhelm von Humboldt, our own Emerson, have all in spirit joined with Goethe in singing that the secret of the highest happiness of man rests in the preservation of his own free personality":

"Hochstes Gluck der Erdenkinder,
Sei nur die Personlichkeit."

Dreamers are constantly devising schemes by which the idle and incompetent may live off the proceeds of the diligent; labor unions deprive their members of the liberty of speech and the liberty of work; socialism would reduce all to a common level; syndicates and trusts break down individual enterprise; sectarian colleges limit their calls to professors who will echo their tenets; and thus in all directions the free growth of the individual is hemmed in by the hedges of prejudice, tradition, creed and false theory.

He liked to take life at right angles. I mean that he was wont to question his friends, or, indeed, chance acquaintances, as to their ideal of life, their purpose in life, and their notion of happiness. It was out of such colloquies that his book upon the Pursuit of Happiness grew, in which the wisdom of a philosophic and observant life is framed into a gospel. In Europe and America he sought the society of anarchists, and mingled sometimes with the malcontents of the world that he might appreciate their grievance and weigh their propositions of reform or change.

In politics Brinton was an ardent patriot. He believed in the immense future of America. His frequent residence abroad never estranged him from his country. His cheerful optimism suffered no eclipse. After America I think his interests were with France. He understood the French people, and he enjoyed French life. His chief friends among foreign Américanistes were in Paris—the Comte de Charency, the Marquis de Nadaillac, and Prince Roland Bonaparte. He was a social creature, a man of cities and of streets, and it was with an unfailing and youthful joy that he returned to Paris to wander

Thro' wind and rain and watch the Seine,
And feel the Boulevard break again
To warmth and light and bliss.

Science has suffered a serious loss in the death of Dr. Brinton, but to his friends the loss is irreparable. He is buried in our hearts. But a little while ago and he moved among us with a firm step and an alert bearing. He seemed so cheerful, so happy, so vigorous and so young. Suddenly that alertness was shaken, and the vital forces swiftly failed. He was spared the "cold gradations of decay." He had lived a blameless, devoted and beneficent life. His work is permanent and valuable. He could say with Landor: "I have warmed both hands before the fire of life. It sinks, and I am ready to depart."

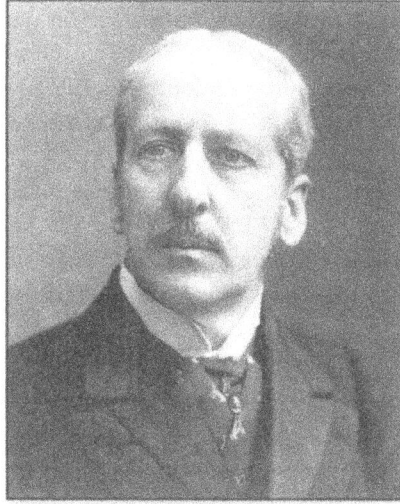

WILLIAM PEPPER JR.

1843–1898 (APS 1870)

Memoir by James Tyson

In the early part of July, 1863, immediately after the battle of Gettysburg, I was in charge of a small military hospital in Harrisburg, Pa., when notified of my appointment as resident physician in the Pennsylvania Hospital. Arriving at the Hospital a few days later, I found among the staff of officers Mr. William Pepper, Jr. Mr. Pepper was then a student of medicine substituting Dr. John Conrad, the Hospital apothecary, who was absent on his vacation. It fell to my lot to be Dr. Pepper's room-mate during his temporary residence in the Hospital, and thus began our friendly relations.

On Friday, the 1st of July, 1898, I had just left my house, and was walking on Spruce street, when Dr. Pepper drove up to the sidewalk, jumped lightly from his carriage and joined me. He announced that he would start for California on the 7th of July, and continued walking with me up Spruce street, chatting gaily and laying plans for the next summer, until Eighteenth street was reached, when he left me with a cheerful, hearty good-by. I never saw him again.

Between these two dates lay just thirty-five years of uninterrupted friendship and exceptionally close intercourse. Brightness, alertness, enthusiasm were the qualities which I recall of him at our first meeting. Cheerfulness, hopefulness, courage—infinite courage, in the light of subsequent events—were conspicuous at our last. These qualities, together with the sweet courtesy which characterized his relations with men and women of all stations are, in a word, a description of his personal life.

The last-named indispensable attribute of true gentleness, courtesy and consideration alike to all, inferiors as well as superiors, was as natural to him as life itself, and was one of the secrets of his influence over men as well as his success as a physician. It is of him as the latter and as a teacher of medicine and author that I have been asked to speak tonight in behalf of my colleagues of the Medical Faculty of the University and of the College of Physicians of Philadelphia.

Dr. Pepper's qualities as a physician were an unusual ability in diagnosis, a power to inspire confidence and by a rare and inimitable manner to cause those who consulted him to feel encouraged and hopeful. His ability in diagnosis was founded on a primary intelligence quickened by a rapidity of thought and comprehension which enabled him almost at a glance to recognize the disturbing causes at work in a sick person.

His method of diagnosis in this respect was very different from that of his father, Dr. William Pepper, who was professor of Medicine in the University when his son and I were students. His method was to make a patient and exhaustive examination of the case, weighing each symptom and physical sign, and, after he had done so, to cautiously draw his conclusions, which were always well founded and rarely changed.

The younger Pepper's diagnosis was more rapid, more brilliant and, though commonly sustained by the autopsy, had sometimes to be altered. I have often been surprised, during consultations with him, at the quickness with which he recognized a morbid condition and the causes leading to it, as well as the consequences which were sure to follow it. For many years a close student of morbid anatomy, it was his habit to conceive the morbid state whence followed naturally the symptoms of the case in hand. On the other hand, Dr. Pepper was not dogmatic in diagnosis. He was keenly alive to the possibility of error and was always ready to admit his mistakes.

More striking even was the second attribute mentioned as a characteristic of Dr. Pepper as a physician, the power to encourage and uplift those who consulted him. This effect was not confined to the sick alone. In fact, no one who knew Dr. Pepper ever failed, at some one time or another, to come under this spell of encouragement and upliftedness. Time and again I have gone to him concerning some one of the matters of our common interest, doubtful and discouraged by the outlook, and after a short interview left him hopeful and light-hearted. So it was with the sick. Hope replaced despair in the heart of the patient, and joy replaced sadness in that of loving relatives and friends. It is needless to say that disappointment and even bitterness sometimes followed because the favorable prognosis was not always realized. Yet no one dare say that this hopefulness was assumed or that any deception was intended. It was the natural outflow of a sanguine spirit, and was a part of that same temperament which caused him to assume and carry to a successful issue large undertakings which others deemed impossible. It did far more good than harm, and many lives were prolonged and hours of agony averted and substituted by the bliss that comes of ignorance.

In prescribing for patients he was not lavish of drugs, and his prescriptions were simple. He was, however, explicit and impressive in direction, so that persons rarely forgot what he ordered. Especially apt was he in the selection of diet, so that he became unusually successful in affections of the stomach and bowels, and acquired an enviable reputation as a specialist in their treatment.

It is impossible to separate Dr. Pepper as a physician from Dr. Pepper as a teacher. From my earliest recollection of him his talks upon medical subjects gave the impression of authority, and any one proposing a new venture in its teaching naturally consulted him. He himself early became an investigator and teacher. On account of his father's delicate health, the younger Pepper did not at once enter a hospital, cheerfully sacrificing to filial duty, opportunities which he, above all others, was qualified to appreciate. On this account he sought for a time to make outdoor dispensary practice substitute the hospital, and worked up his cases in a thorough way which any one else would have deemed impossible, indeed would scarcely have thought of. I substituted for him and followed him in some of this work, and had a good opportunity of learning his methods.

Later, after his father's death, which occurred in 1864, he entered the Pennsylvania Hospital as resident physician, and served eighteen months, from April, 1865, to October, 1866. This latter course was the natural result of his enthusiasm in medicine and a determination to secure the best possible foundation. Many men, having once launched upon practice, would have thought it too great a sacrifice to go back to the beginning, and start, as it were, afresh. While at the Hospital, he was an enthusiastic worker. One could rarely enter his room without finding him peering into the microscope or dissecting out an aneurysm or some other morbid product of the autopsy.

He was appointed Curator of the Pathological Museum of the Pennsylvania Hospital March 26, 1866, and served until September 28, 1870. During this time he prepared a descriptive catalogue of the pathological specimens in the Museum numbering 138 closely printed octavo pages, based on one previously written by Dr. Thomas G. Morton.

His teaching began with that of morbid anatomy in a course delivered at the Pennsylvania Hospital while Curator in 1867. He did not, however, give more than two courses at the Hospital, because the institution of an autumn course of lectures at the University of Pennsylvania, in 1868, led to his appointment as lecturer on this same subject, morbid anatomy.

His election in 1867 as one of the visiting physicians to the Philadelphia Hospital (Blockley) gave him the first opportunity to lecture to large classes, and he quickly became popular as a clinical teacher. In 1870 he was appointed lecturer on Clinical Medicine in the University, and became professor of Clinical Medicine in 1876. In this year also he was appointed Medical Director of the Centennial Exposition, and received from the King of Sweden the decoration of Knight Commander of the Order of St. Olaf in recognition of his distinguished services.

In 1884 he succeeded Prof. Alfred Still as professor of the Theory and Practice of Medicine and Clinical Medicine and held this chair until his death, July 28, 1898. During thirteen years of this period, 1881 to 1894, he was also Provost of the University. His greatest ability was shown in teaching clinical medicine. He attracted students and patients from all parts of the country, and his Saturday clinics were often made up of cases who had thus come to seek his opinion. He never hesitated to take up any case, however difficult, and generally succeeded in unfolding it to the edification of the class and satisfaction of the patient.

In didactic teaching, though attractive, he was less conspicuously successful. Latterly his numerous engagements made a thorough preparation of his lectures impossible, and led at times to a diffuseness which weakened their force and emphasis. His readiness at speaking favored this, and he has told me that this very facility of speech which served him so often and so well was really a disadvantage to him. Graceful and easy in manner, yet dignified and totally without vulgar oratorial effort, his pleasant voice, distinct utterance and great command of language made his speech truly silvern.

Dr. Pepper's conception of the office of the medical teacher was a very broad one. He would have him broadly educated in letters and arts as well as learned in medicine, an associate of men and interested in public enterprises—in a word, a man of affairs, not a mere pedagogue in the narrower sense of the term. He considered that it was the teacher's privilege and duty to take an active part in the management of his College or University and his own life was an exemplification of his ideal.

Dr. Pepper cannot be considered as a teacher of medicine from the standpoint of the lecturer only. As a writer he taught many more than as a lecturer. It would, however, be impossible to treat of him as an author except in the most superficial manner in the short time allotted me. With the preparation of his thesis, which was commenced in the summer of our residence at the Pennsylvania Hospital referred to, began a long series of practical papers published chiefly in the Proceedings of the Pathological Society, the American Journal of the Medical Sciences, The Medical and Surgical Reporter, The Medical Times, which he founded in 1870, and edited for two years; The Medical News, and finally the Philadelphia Medical Journal, which also owes its existence to him.

His first paper of importance was on "The Fluorescence of Tissues," and appeared in the first volume of the Pennsylvania Hospital Reports in 1868. It was prepared in conjunction with his friend, Dr. Edward Rhoads, and involved much physical and chemical research. Its object was to show that a substance found in the normal tissues by Bence Jones, which possessed a property of fluorescence like quinine and called by him "animal quinoidine," disappeared under the influence of the malarial poison.

Another paper of great value published in the same volume of the Pennsylvania Hospital Reports was "On the Morphological Changes of the Blood in Malarial Fever," by Dr. J. Forsyth Meigs, assisted by Dr. Edward Rhoads and Dr. Pepper. The article was based on the study of 123 cases of a severe form of bilious fever with six deaths which occurred in the service of Dr. Meigs at the Pennsylvania Hospital during the summer of 1865, while Dr. Pepper and Dr. Rhoads were resident physicians. All the details of the study were made by Dr. Pepper and Dr. Rhoads, and involved an enormous amount of microscopical investigation.

Among the more important subjects treated in this earlier part of his career were "Phosphorus Poisoning," American Journal of the Medical Sciences, in 1869; "Variola," ibid., 1869; "Tracheotomy in Chronic Laryngitis," Philadelphia Medical Times, 1870; "Abdominal Tumors," ibid., 1870; "Trephining in Cerebral Disease," American Journal of the Medical Sciences, 1871; "Progressive Muscular Sclerosis, or, Hypertrophic Muscular Paralysis," Philadelphia Medical Times, 1871; "Local Treatment of Tuberculous Cavities in the Lungs," American Journal of the Medical Sciences, 1874; "Operative and Treatment of Pleural Effusions," Philadelphia Medical Times, 1874; "Progressive Pernicious Anaemia,"" American Journal of the Medical Sciences, 1875; "Addison's Disease and Its Relations to Anaematoses," ibid., 1877; "Appendicitis," Transactions of the Medical Society of Pennsylvania, 1876.

The papers on "Progressive Pernicious Anaemia," and "Addison's Disease" were exhaustive and up to date of publication. In the former he suggested the name of "Anaematosis," which has been acknowledged by Hermann Eichhorst and Thomas Clifford Albutt. The paper on "Appendicitis" was also a valuable one, his experience having been large and his studies among the first important contributions to the subject.

Among his more recent papers was a contribution to the "Climatological Study of Phthisis in Pennsylvania," read before the Climatological Association at its third annual session in 1886. It was a methodical and exhaustive investigation into the territorial distribution of consumption in the State of Pennsylvania, and of its causes, illustrated by elaborate maps showing the peculiarities of soil and climate of each county, and must be the basis of all future investigations into the same subject in the State of Pennsylvania.

Of his larger works, his edition of the late Dr. John Forsythe Meigs' book on Diseases of Children, published in 1870, came first. The book was largely rewritten by him and much enlarged, so that it was properly renamed, Meigs and Pepper on Diseases of Children. It was for years the standard text-book on this subject in this country, and was highly esteemed in England.

"A System of Medicine by American Authors, 1885–6", a treatise in five large octavo volumes, was edited by Dr. Pepper. He did not personally contribute many articles, but two of the most important, that on "Catarrhal Pneumonia" and that on "Relapsing Fever," were written by him and will come to be regarded among medical classics.

He had unusual opportunities for the study of relapsing fever in the epidemic which prevailed in Philadelphia in 1879, and his paper is perhaps the most valuable ever written on the subject by an American. "Pepper's System," as it is called, became at once the recognized authority in all diseases prevalent in this country and many thousand copies were sold in a very short time. Its success was also largely due to the signal ability shown in the selection of collaborators. No similar work published in this country included so brilliant an array of authors. Every one was anxious to enlist under his banner and no one declined.

His latest work was a Text-book of Medicine, by different authors. It consisted of two large octavo volumes, was published in 1893-1894, and had a large sale among students and physicians.

Dr. Pepper's addresses, of which he made many on medical subjects, were always happy and among the most effective of his efforts. I well remember the impression made by one of the earliest of these, the "Address in Medicine," before the Pennsylvania State Medical Society at its meeting in Pottsville in 1875, when he was but thirty years old. Full of practical information, clearly and impressively read, it was the most refreshing event of the meeting. The older members of the Society were enthusiastic over it, and it won him many admirers.

His two addresses, "Higher Medical Education the True Interest of the Public and of the Profession," read before the Medical Department of the University of Pennsylvania, were admirable examples of his power in this direction, The first was delivered October 1, 1877, on the occasion of the change of curriculum from two to three years, and the second sixteen years later, on October 2, 1893, at the inauguration of the four-year course of medical study. They abound in important and interesting information, including statistical data of great value, attractively and forcibly presented.

To be eloquent on subjects connected with medicine is very difficult, well-nigh impossible, and yet in his presidential address before the first Pan-American Medical Congress, in Washington, September, 1893, Dr. Pepper held in rapt attention a large and promiscuous audience. Its subject was "The State of this Continent and its Aboriginal Inhabitants at the time of its discovery by Columbus, and the obstacles which opposed him and the great men who completed his work" together with "The state of Medical Science in Europe at the time of the discovery and the spirit which controlled its subsequent course." Like the two University addresses alluded to, it abounds in valuable information involving laborious historical research gathered and collated at a time when he was excessively busy. It excited the enthusiastic admiration of the representatives from British and Spanish America, and from South America and Mexico, which was reflected in the reception given to him in the city of Mexico at the second triennial meeting of this Congress in 1896, and in the memorial meeting held in the city of Mexico since his death.

The Pan-American Congress itself is a permanent monument of his ability as an organizer. At its inception he had few sympathizers, but like all else he undertook he made the Washington meeting a magnificent success, and the two splendid volumes of nearly 1200 pages each, which contain the transactions published in English and Spanish, abundantly attest it. They include a vast amount of information bearing on medicine from all parts of North and South America, which could in no other way have been accumulated. He was ably seconded in the organization of the Congress by Dr. Charles A. Reed, of Cincinnati, the Secretary General.

Dr. Pepper took a warm interest in the medical societies of the city and country. As has been the case with so many of the medical men of Philadelphia, who obtained distinction, the Pathological Society was the arena in which he first availed himself of opportunity. He became a member in 1865, and was for a long time the most energetic and active of its members. The Transactions abound in reports of specimens presented by him, eighty-four in all, in a comparatively short time, and in remarks made by him on specimens exhibited by others. He was made Vice-President in 1870, and President from 1873 to 1876.

He became a member of the Philadelphia County Medical Society in 1871, and of the Medical Society of the State of Pennsylvania in 1875, and in the early part of his career was a frequent contributor to their Proceedings. His proposition for membership to the County Medical Society was signed by Drs. Alfred Stillé, Augustus H. Fish and Charles S. Boker. The first is still living. The last two preceded Dr. Pepper in death.

He was one of the founders of the Obstetrical Society of Philadelphia in 1869. He was chairman of the Committee of Arrangements of the American Medical Association when the latter met in Philadelphia, in 1876. At the annual meeting of this Association, held at Newport, R.I., in June, 1888, he read an impressive sketch of Dr. Benjamin Rush, and became thus the instrument of numerous subscriptions made on the spot to the Rush Monument Fund.

He was a member of the American Neurological and Climatological Societies, and one of the founders (1886) of the Association of American Physicians, a society then limited to one hundred of the physicians of the United States and Canada, and was its President in 1891. Another one of the numerous monuments to his ability as an organizer is the Triennial Congress of American Physicians and Surgeons. Although he was not the originator of this association—this distinction resting with the late Dr. Claudius Mastin, of Mobile, Ala., Dr. Pepper was chairman of the first Executive Committee, and skillfully guided this body to a successful organization of the Congress, and he made an able address at the opening meeting in Washington, September 18, 1889.

Dr. Pepper was elected a Fellow of the College of Physicians in 1867, and immediately took an active interest in its proceedings. His most important papers were "Trephining in Cerebral Disease," read May 18, 1870; "The Internal Use of Nitrate of Silver," read May 7, 1877; and "Addison's Disease," read January 7, 1886. In addition to these papers, his remarks on the communications of other Fellows were always full of valuable information gained from his reading and rapidly growing experiences.

Thus succeeding a paper read by Dr. J. Ewing Mears, June 2, 1875, "On Encysted Dropsy of the Peritoneum," although Dr. Pepper had been only eleven years in practice, he cited three cases of the rare condition of encysted dropsy of the abdomen which had occurred in his practice. And thus it was with every subject which came up when he happened to be present.

In consequence of the exacting demands on his time by the numerous and important interests in which he was concerned of late years, he was compelled, much to his personal regret, to neglect the meetings of the College, but he always took a warm interest and I know looked forward to the time when, freed of some of his responsibilities, he might again contribute to its proceedings and take a hand in its management. It was through his instrumentality chiefly that, a number of years ago, about 1870, the College for a time increased its meetings to two a month, with the idea that one meeting should be devoted to scientific matters only, and the other to business. At that day, however, the number of Fellows was much smaller and there was much less activity among them, so that the semi-monthly meetings could not be maintained. Quite recently when it appeared to some of us that the time had come for the formation of a section in medicine for the purpose of stimulating this department, Dr. Pepper attended the meeting for organization, in January, 1897, though he was at the time overwhelmed with work, and had not for a long time attended a similar meeting. This was the last meeting of a Medical Society he ever attended.

For several years prior to 1898, Philadelphia was without a first-class weekly medical journal. Dr. Pepper, always alive to the interests of Philadelphia in all directions, felt that this was a serious drawback to the position the city had always held in medical affairs, and decided that it must not continue. Early in the fall of 1897, he began to organize a company for the purpose of establishing such a journal, and, with his usual sagacity, he sought to interest not a single school of medicine only, but all the schools in Philadelphia, as well as the profession at large. But more than this, he did what had never been done before. He succeeded in interesting prominent business men other than publishers of medical books, including those of large experience in the management of successful newspapers.

By the 1st of October, 1897, the arrangements were completed, a Board of Trustees organized, and Dr. George M. Gould appointed editor, with an Executive Committee representing all interests, to aid him. On Saturday, January 1, 1898, appeared the first number of the Philadelphia Medical Journal, which has already established itself in the front rank of the medical journals of the world, and adds another to the many results of Dr. Pepper's public spirit and energy.

Dr. Pepper was an easy, clear and forcible writer as he was a speaker. He had excellent command of the resources of the language and was never at a loss for appropriate and well-chosen words to express himself. He was at all times too busy a man to devote time to the evolution of ornately expressed thought or sentiment, but what he wrote was always interesting and neatly expressed. It is really necessary to go back to some of his earlier writings to appreciate the possibilities of his style in this direction. In the memoir of his dear friend, Edward Rhoads, read before the College of Physicians, February 7, 1871, will be found a sentiment which is as appropriate to this occasion as it was on that of the loving tribute to his friend. It is as follows:

"The wheels of human life and action revolve ceaselessly, and place a rapidly increasing distance between us and any passing event. Each day's cares and activity throng the mind, and dim the images of the past that memory seeks to cherish, until the joy or sorrow that for the time filled the whole life seems in but a few months only the shadowy phantom of some far-distant experience."

"It is true, moreover, that in a life so full and overfull of thought and action as that of the present day, there is but little leisure left to devote to the contemplation of the future, and far less to spend in reflection on the past. Whatever the past has made us, we are; whatever it has given to us, we hold and strive to make the means of securing more and more; but of what it has taken from us, we rarely think, but turn impatiently from the sorrowful reminiscences which sometimes stir in the depths of our being, muttering, "Let the dead past bury its dead." To a great extent this is needful, if we are to advance in our work actively and hopefully. But do we not often carry this too far, and in struggling manfully against the depression and despondency which follow a great grief, often end in not only throwing off these, but also in forgetting and losing much of the sweetness and usefulness which might always remain with us?"

"That with his talents, his education, his opportunities and his energy, Dr. Pepper should have accomplished all he did as a physician, a teacher of medicine and medical writer is not strange. Others have perhaps done as much. But that he should have accomplished thus much and as much more as he did in the thirty-five short years of his active life is truly marvelous. The measure of what he accomplished outside the part allotted me to consider will appear from others before the evening has closed, but I may be permitted to sum up by saying that what he accomplished made him easily what he was at the date of his too early death—Philadelphia's first and foremost citizen."

EDITORS' NOTE

Dr. Tyson's memoir of William Pepper Jr. characterizes him as a successful practitioner and teacher of medicine leaving additional aspects of his record to other speakers. These speakers included the governor, the mayor and representatives of the many institutions in which Dr. Pepper played a founding or dominant role. Their tributes to him as a visionary University executive and civic leader occupied an additional 55 pages and are summarized here only briefly. They substantiate Dr. Tyson's concluding sentence, that at the time of his death Dr. Pepper was his City's "first and foremost citizen." As a civic leader Pepper founded or was the dominant force and often the financial benefactor in establishing the City's Free Public Library System, the Commercial Museum The Museum of Archaeology and Paleontology and the Wistar Institute of Anatomy and Biology.

In addition William Pepper Jr. may have been the most important figure in the history of both the University of Pennsylvania and its School of Medicine. In the early 1870s, though only a junior faculty member Dr. Pepper was the strongest and most effective advocate of establishing a site for patient based instruction by building a teaching hospital, the nation's first to be owned and controlled by a University. Through fund raising from his friends, family and the State Legislature he accomplished this in 1874 and soon became the unofficial head of the new hospital. Then within 4 years over strong opposition from entrenched senior faculty he was largely responsible for changing Penn's outdated, inadequate medical school course by extending it from two years to three years and by introducing a full time system for the professors. Later while he was University Provost (1881–1894) Pepper further extended the medical school to 4 years. He also prevented matriculation of unqualified students by instituting entrance examinations or other requirements. In 1892 he endowed the Pepper Laboratory for clinical testing and research, naming it for his father. The Hopkins dean William Welch described this as a unique resource which should become mandatory for all teaching hospitals.

At the time Dr. Pepper occupied the post, the Provost rather than the President was the ranking executive of the University. According to Martin Myerson Provost Pepper used this power to awaken Penn from what he said had been a "state of slumber" since the time of Benjamin Franklin. He transformed a parochial institution compromised of a few loosely connected departments into a major U.S. university with a research as well as teaching mission.

During his 13 years as Provost Pepper established for the University two new libraries and 15 new departments, divisions and schools including: The Department of Finance and Economy (the Wharton School), The Department of Philosophy, The Department of Veterinary Medicine, The Department of Biology, The Department of Physical Education, The Department of Archaeology and Paleontology, The Department of Hygiene, The Graduate Department for Women, The School of Architecture and The School for Nurses.

William Pepper Jr. was only one of six APS members from the Pepper family which for almost a century was remarkably influential. The dominance their family had over the University of Pennsylvania's School of Medicine for 3 generations led to the attachment of a dynastic authority to the Peppers. The first William Pepper as Professor of Medicine signed his son's diploma; William Pepper Jr. as Professor of Medicine and Provost of the University signed his son's diploma and the third William Pepper as Dean and Professor of Medicine signed the diploma of his son Sergeant Pepper. The youngest son of William Pepper Jr., Oliver Hazard Perry Pepper, graduated from medical school after his father's death thus missing his father's signature on his diploma but nevertheless he too became a Professor of Medicine.

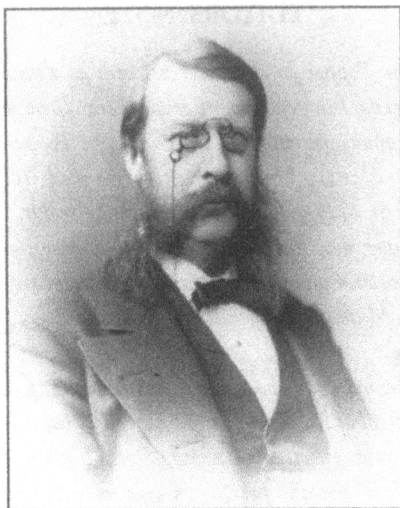

GEORGE FREDERICK BARKER

1835–1910 (APS 1873)

Memoir by Elihu Thomson

Dr. Barker was born July 14, 1835, at Charlestown, Mass., and attended school there, afterwards going to Berwick and Yarmouth academies in Maine, and to Lawrence Academy in Groton, Mass. When about sixteen he entered as apprentice the establishment of J. M. Wightman in Boston, a maker of philosophical instruments, and remained there five years. This apprentice period must have given a training very valuable to one who was afterward to so freely use scientific apparatus. After taking the degree of Bachelor of Philosophy at the Sheffield Scientific School, where he was also assistant to Professor Silliman, he entered the Harvard Medical School as a student and assistant in chemistry.

From this time his career as a science teacher and lecturer was continued with but little interruption. He received the degree of Doctor of Medicine from the Albany Medical College in 1863, having completed his medical course there while Acting Professor of Chemistry in the school. In 1864 he served as professor of natural sciences in the Western University of Pennsylvania, soon thereafter going to Yale as demonstrator in the medical department, where in 1867 he was appointed Professor of Physiological Chemistry and Toxicology, a chair which he held for six years, when he was appointed Professor of Physics in the University of Pennsylvania. Beginning in 1873 he continued this work as head of the department for twenty-seven years, becoming Professor Emeritus in 1900.

Before coming to Philadelphia he had acted as State Chemist in Connecticut, giving testimony in some noted cases of poisoning. He was also at times engaged as expert in patent cases, concerning electric lighting, telephones, batteries and chemical processes. It was when Dr. Barker took the chair of physics in the University of Pennsylvania that the writer first had the privilege of his acquaintance. He was then among the faithful attendants upon the meetings of the American Philosophical Society, of which he became a member in 1873 and later, as is well known, served as an officer of the Society, acting as Secretary from 1877 to 1897, and also Vice-President, between 1890 and 1908.

The record of the scientific work of Dr. Barker is distinguished by remarkable versatility. Moreover, his temper of mind was such that, while giving full worth to research in so-called pure science, he did not lose sight of the practical application of scientific principles as a most important factor in human progress. As a chemist he dealt ably with the purely theoretical side of chemical problems, yet was an eminent and trusted practical chemist. He gave a large fraction of his life's work to abstract physical science, but was ever keenly interested in engineering.

Nor did he fail in extending this interest to other branches of science besides those which he had made peculiarly his own. We find him observing transits and solar eclipses, and making and recording observations in astronomy with the same ability and enthusiasm which he manifested in chemistry or physics. Even in his later years we find the same acute interest in his studies and work in Roentgen rays and radio-activity. It was also true that at all times he showed for the work of others a generous appreciation and interest, and when such work commended itself to him he was not slow in assisting towards its proper recognition.

In the early Philadelphia days Dr. Barker lectured frequently in public to large and appreciative audiences. He spared no pains to interest and instruct those who attended. Was there a new development or discovery in science, he strove to make his auditors appreciate it as he did. His mechanical and practical skill was of great aid in devising and arranging apt and often brilliant experimental illustrations, with which his popular lectures were crowded.

It was the writer's privilege as a young man to be present on a number of such occasions at the Academy of Music, and he remembers vividly a lecture on electric lighting in which, as a unique feature, an early Gramme dynamo, secured from abroad by Dr. Barker, was driven by a gas engine, and used to furnish the electrical current. Before that time a large voltaic battery, almost prohibitive from its cumbersomeness and cost, would have been required to produce any semblance of the brilliant effects of the electric arc then shown. This was at a time when there was but little appreciation of the possible great future growth of electric lighting and about two years before the invention of the incandescent lamp by Edison.

As a natural result, however, we find that Dr. Barker was not only, from the first, in personal touch with Edison in his pioneer work, but was one of those deeply interested in his early incandescent lamp development. More broadly it can be said that throughout his long service to science, Dr. Barker followed with special ardor the rapid and important growth of electrical science which has continued in the intervening years.

When the American Philosophical Society celebrated the 150th anniversary of its foundation, it was he who, under the title of "Electrical Progress Since 1743," studiously reviewed the advance of electrical science due to workers such as Franklin, Faraday, Hare, Henry and others. As another evidence not only of his deep interest in electrical advancement but of the early recognition of his foremost position at the time, he was appointed U.S. Commissioner to the Paris Electrical Exposition held in 1881, and an official delegate to the Electrical Congress then held. This was indeed a famous congress, by which much work of vital interest and importance was either accomplished or initiated, particularly concerning the nomenclature of the several electrical units, and the evaluation of standards; a work which has been continued by the subsequent international chambers of delegates at each of the important Congresses held since that time; the last being that at St. Louis in 1904.

At the Paris Exposition of 1881, which was the first exposition to be devoted to electricity solely, Dr. Barker was also made vice-president of the Jury of Awards, and in recognition of his services received the decoration of Commander de la Legion D'Honneur, an honor accorded to but few Americans. He was also a member of the U.S. Commission at the Electrical Congress held during the Philadelphia Electrical Exhibition of the Franklin Institute in 1884. He served also on the Jury of Awards at the World's Columbian Exposition in 1893.

During his long connection with the University of Pennsylvania, his services were valued very highly by his associates; he was always helpful in the solution of the problems presented, and brought to bear a ripe judgment so as to decide upon the course to be taken in any case with fairness and calmness. His service to the community was none the less valuable. This was evident in his work while a member of the Board of Public Education, and his counsel in relation to such matters as water supply, illuminating gas and other municipal problems was much esteemed.

Dr. Barker was one of the first to point out the fallacies and trickery of the famous Keely motor scheme, and to denounce it in the public prints. This scheme was actively exploited in the late seventies in Philadelphia. Needless is it to say that all the subsequent history of that long-lived fraud, and its final wind-up and exposure upon the death of Keely amply confirmed the entire justice of Dr. Barker's original denunciation of it.

As an author and writer he was, as in other things, most careful and conscientious. His text-book on "Elementary Chemistry" which first appeared in 1870 went through many editions, and was esteemed as embodying the most advanced thought, presented for the first time in our language thoroughly and systematically. No less an authority than Wolcott Gibbs commended the book highly.

Barker's "Physics, Advanced Course" published in 1892 as one of the American Science Series, was likewise an embodiment of the most modern views and met with a hearty reception. The treatment was mainly from the standpoint of energy and interchanges therein, and the ether of space was frankly assumed as the fundamental thing in dealing with all forms of radiation.

From his habit of mind it was to be expected that in his scientific papers we should also find the results of the latest investigations. He was particular in giving a comprehensive bibliography of the subject, where it was possible. Thus, the valuable address delivered by him before the Chemical Society at Columbia University in March, 1903, is a model paper. Its subject was "Radio-Activity and Chemistry," and its great historical value will be understood when it is stated that to it is appended a bibliography of no less than ninety titles of papers by the leading investigators.

Some of his earlier papers and addresses assisted to a considerable degree in enforcing the great principles of conservation and correlation of forces, the discussion of which was carried on actively in the period between 1860 and 1880. Before those years the ideas of permanence of energy and the importance of energy interchanges had not received universal recognition or acceptance. It is now generally recognized that the indestructibility of energy is a more necessary postulate than the indestructibility of matter.

Dr. Barker's logical mind did not limit itself to the consideration of physical forces merely. He had taken the degree of doctor of medicine and it was natural that he should be led to consider the relations between the physical and so-called vital forces. We find his views expressed in a paper entitled "The Correlation of Vital and Physical Forces," published in 1875 by Van Nostrand, and also in his address as retiring president of the American Association for the Advancement of Science, at the Boston meeting in 1882. This latter address was entitled "Some Modern Aspects of the Life

Question." He identifies vital force or energy as that stored in the complex protoplasm under physical and chemical conditions only; a view which more and more guides the biochemists of today in their researches.

The Association address is an excellent example of clear logical scientific thinking. In it Dr. Barker drew ably from his rich fund of knowledge in physics, chemistry, biology, and kindred branches. He claims for science its true position as interpreter of the things which can be known, but points out clearly the limitations of this knowledge.

The writer may be pardoned formaking a few quotations:

"But the properties of bodies are only the characters by which we differentiate them. Two bodies having the same properties would only be two portions of the same substance. Because life, therefore, is unlike other properties of matter, it by no means follows that it is not a property of matter. No dictum is more absolute in science than the one which predicates properties upon constitution. To say that this property exhibited by protoplasm, marvelous and even unique though it be, is not a natural result of the constitution of matter itself, but is due to an unknown entity, a tertium quid which inhabits and controls it, is opposed to all scientific analogy and experience. To the statement of the vitalist that there is no evidence that life is a property of matter, we may reply with emphasis that there is not the slightest proof that it is not."

Again, at the close of the address, speaking of the dependence of all activity on the earth upon solar radiation:

"It is a beautiful conception of science which regards the energy which is manifested on the earth as having its origin in the sun. Pulsating awhile in the ether, the molecules of which fill the intervening space, this motion reaches our earth and communicates its tremor to the molecules of matter. Instantly all starts into life. The winds move, the waters rise and fall, the lightnings flash and the thunders roll, all as subdivisions of this received power."

And further:

"But all this energy is only a transitory possession. As the sunlight gilds the mountain top and then glances off into space, so this energy touches upon and beautifies our earth and then speeds on its way. What other worlds it reaches and vivifies, we may never know. Beyond the veil of the seen, science may not penetrate. But religion, more hopeful, seeks there for the new heavens and the new earth wherein shall be solved the problems of a higher life."

That the taking up of the teaching of physics by Dr. Barker did not prevent a continued interest in chemical studies is shown by his serving as the chairman of the sub-section of chemistry of the American Association in 1876, when he delivered a notable address on "The Molecule and the Atom." In this he points out the importance of considering the energy interchanges in chemical reactions, a matter which up to that time had been more or less neglected.

Even as late as 1891, he was honored by being made president of the American Chemical Society, and delivered an address on the "Borderland between Physics and Chemistry," in which he deals with the necessity for distinguishing the fundamental notion of "mass" from that of "weight." He further showed the rich harvest to be expected in the application of the kinetic theory to solutions, and concluded by a remarkably clear exposition of what was then known of the nature of electric forces in their relation to chemical actions.

In these later years, it has indeed been the field of physical chemistry which has yielded an abundant harvest; the advances in it have been of the greatest importance to science. Indeed, the electro-physicist of today has even split the one time ultimate chemical atom into the more fundamental electrons. We must credit Dr. Barker with a keen appreciation of the directions in which further scientific advances were to be made.

None the less clear was his prevision of the future of applied science. In this connection the writer must content himself by quoting from a brief paper read at the Saratoga Meeting of the American Association for the Advancement of Science in 1879. The title of the paper was "On the Conversion of Mechanical energy into Heat by Dynamo Electric Machines." It must be remembered that at the time the paper was read no practical incandescent electric lamp had been made, and industrial electric development had scarcely begun even with the older arc light. The quotation reads:

"The amount of heat actually obtainable from dynamo electric machines when worked upon a commercial scale, is a question which in the near future is to become of very considerable commercial importance. That electric distribution, at least in our larger cities, is ultimately to be the source of light supply, is already placed beyond a peradventure. But far more than a simple light production is to be expected of this marvelous agent. It must not only light our houses, but it must warm them and must furnish mechanical power to them for a thousand petty operations now either done not at all, or done by manual labor. It must pump the water, raise the elevator, run the sewing machine, turn the spit, perform its part of the laundry service, **and perhaps even assist in the cooking.**"

As before indicated, it was natural that the early work of Edison on the carbon filament lamp should greatly interest Dr. Barker. This lamp was not brought out until 1880, but we find that it was in that year tested as a light source by him, acting in collaboration with Professor Henry A. Rowland. The results were published in the American Journal of Science, and in the Chemical News. This account of early tests was followed in 1881 by papers dealing with the general subject of electric light photometry and by results of tests.

Dr. Barker was chairman of the Sub-commission on Incandescent Lamps at the Paris Electrical Exposition in 1881, the other members being Wm. Crookes, E. Hagenbach, A. Kundt and E. Mascart. There is no need to make any comment on the standing of these men. Their work was in fact pioneer work done at the start of an industry which today has become one of immense importance. As the Paris Exposition of 1881 was the first to be devoted entirely to electricity and its applications, it possessed a peculiar interest. The International Congress of Electricians held at the same time has been before referred to. Dr. Barker prepared a report on the proceedings of this congress.

A glance at the list of writings of Dr. Barker will show at once the great range of subjects about which he had informed himself, and upon which he was equipped to accomplish valuable scientific work. His alertness of mind, even a few years before his death, is plainly evident in his later papers on such subjects as radioactivity and intra-atomic energy in 1903, and before that time in his discussion of liquefied air, Roentgen rays, wireless telegraphy, monatomic gases, etc.

It was only to be expected that one so able and active as he was should become the recipient of many honors. Besides those already mentioned, including positions of honor on important commissions and the like, he was given the honorary degree of Doctor of Science by the University of Pennsylvania in 1898, and in the same year, the degree of Doctor of Laws from Allegheny College and also from McGill University. He was elected a member of the National Academy of Sciences in 1876 and later an honorary member of the Royal Institution of Great Britain. He was also a member of scientific societies in France and Germany.

He attended many notable educational and scientific meetings as a delegate from societies or from the University which he so long served. He was assistant editor of the American Journal of Science, from 1868 to 1900, and contributed for a number of years accounts of the year's progress in physics, to the annual Smithsonian Reports. Dr. Barker was married in 1861 to Mary M. Treadway, of New Haven, who survives him, and had five children, of whom three daughters are living. He was in his seventy-fifth year when he died in Philadelphia, last May.

Thus closed a life of great and varied service, one devoted to high ideals—a striking example of industry and achievement, a life spent in doing good. Thus ended the career of a lifelong student of science of an exceptional range of accomplishment, an excellent teacher, and a man of noblest aspirations. To those who knew him well there remains the vivid remembrance of his sterling worth and fine personal qualities.

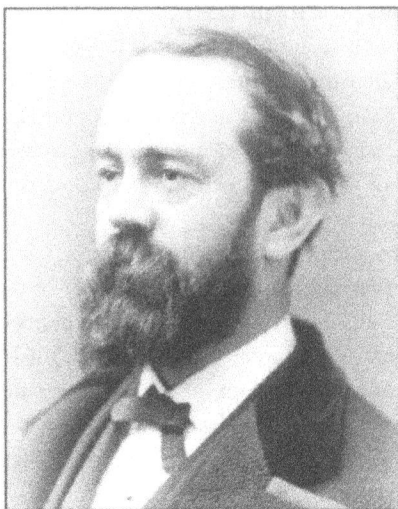

HENRY DRAPER

1837–1882 (APS 1877)

Memoir by George F. Barker

Henry Draper was born on the 7th of March, 1837, in Prince Edward county, Va., his father being at the time Professor of Chemistry and Natural Philosophy in Hampden-Sidney College. When but two years old, his father was called to the chair of Chemistry in the University of the City of New York, and removed to that city in 1839. Henry was entered as a regular scholar, first in the primary, and subsequently in the preparatory schools connected with the University, and at the age of fifteen entered the collegiate department as an undergraduate. Upon the completion of his sophomore year, however, he abandoned the classical course and entered the medical department, from which he graduated with distinction in 1858.

The following year he spent in Europe. While abroad he was elected on the medical staff of Bellevue Hospital; and on his return he assumed the position and discharged its duties for eighteen months. In 1860, at the age of 23, he was elected Professor of Physiology in the Classical department of the University, and, in 1866, to the same chair in the Medical department; being soon after appointed Dean. In 1873, he severed his connection with the medical department; and in 1882, upon the death of his father, he was elected Professor of Chemistry in the Classical department; a position which he held until the close of the current academic year.

Reared in direct contact with science and scientific thought, as Dr. Draper was, it is not surprising that at an early age he developed a decided preference for scientific pursuits. His father was a man not only of the widest scientific knowledge, but he was also of exceptional ability as an investigator. To live in contact with this genial and learned man, was of itself a scientific education of the highest type. Henry was early taken into his confidence in scientific matters, and was called upon to assist his father not only in his lectures, but also in his investigations.

The scientific spirit which presses forward unflaggingly in the pursuit of truth and which wrests from Nature the profoundest secrets by patient and long continued application, had long been characteristic of the elder Draper; it was now fully developed in his son. While yet a medical student, he undertook a most difficult research upon the functions of the spleen; and, conscious of the inaccuracies incident to drawings, he illustrated this research—afterward published as his graduating thesis—with micro-photographs of rare perfection for those early days, all taken by himself. While engaged with the microscope in making these photographs, he discovered that palladious chloride had a remarkable power in darkening or intensifying negatives; an observation subsequently of much value in photography.

During his sojourn in Europe, he had visited the great reflecting telescope of Lord Rosse at Parsonstown, Ireland. The sight of this instrument inspired him with a desire to construct one like it, though on a smaller scale, and turned his attention toward astronomy and astronomical photography. Soon after his return he began the construction of a metal speculum, fifteen inches in diameter, completing it in 1860. Subsequently he accepted a suggestion contained in a letter written to his father by Sir John Herschel, and abandoned speculum metal for silvered glass.

In the year 1861, he made several mirrors of silvered glass, 15-1/2 inches in diameter. The best of these was mounted as a Newtonian telescope, in a small wooden observatory erected at Hastings-on-Hudson, his father's country seat. The details of grinding, polishing, silvering, testing and mounting this reflector, all of which he did with his own hands, were published as a monograph by the Smithsonian Institution. This publication has had a deserved popularity, and has become the standard authority on the subject.

Much experimental work was done with this telescope; that which is best known, being his photograph of the moon. More than 1500 original negatives were taken with this instrument. They were one and a quarter inches in diameter, but such was the perfection of their detail that they bore enlargement to three feet, and in one case to fifty inches without injury.

The success of this mirror stimulated him to undertake a still larger one, and in 1870, he finished a silvered glass mirror, twenty-eight inches in diameter. A new dome was built for it by the side of the old one, the mounting being equatorial, and the telescope Cassegrainian; though subsequently a plane secondary mirror was substituted for the convex one. A refracting telescope of five inches aperture was attached to the tube of the reflector, as a finder. With this larger instrument, work was at once begun upon photographic spectra; and, in 1872, a beautiful photograph was obtained of the spectrum of a Lyrae (Vega), which showed the dark lines; a step far in advance of anything which had been accomplished in this direction up to that time.

Desiring to make simultaneous eye-observations, Dr. Draper, in 1875, placed upon the same axis, a refracting telescope of twelve inches aperture, made by Alvan Clark & Sons. In 1880, this was exchanged for another refractor by the same makers, of eleven and a half inches aperture, but furnished with an additional lens to serve as a photographic corrector.

The work of stellar spectrum photography went steadily on, the new refractor now doing the principal work. More than a hundred such photographs were made, most of these having upon the same plate a photograph of the spectrum of Jupiter, Venus, or the moon. These latter, giving the solar lines by reflection, enabled the stellar lines to be identified by direct comparison.

Reflecting on the extreme sensitiveness of the dry-plate process in photography, he was led to experiment on the reproduction of nebulae by its means; and on the 20th of September, 1880, he succeeded by an exposure of fifty-seven minutes in obtaining a photograph of the nebula in Orion. Satisfied now that the idea was an entirely feasible one, he devoted himself uninterruptedly to securing the greatest possible perfection in the driving clock and to improving the details of manipulation.

In March, 1881, a second and much superior photograph of this nebula was secured after an exposure of 104 minutes. And finally, a year later, on the 14th of March, 1882, he succeeded in making a successful exposure of 137 minutes, and in producing a most superb photograph, which showed stars of the 13.7 magnitude, invisible to the eye, and in which the faint outlying regions of the nebula itself were clearly and beautifully shown. This unrivaled photograph, by far the most brilliant success yet achieved by celestial photography, will ever have a very high astronomical value, since by a comparison with it of photographs of this nebula, taken many years subsequently, changes which are going on in it may be traced and their history written.

Ordinarily the photograph of a spectrum is more difficult than one of the object itself. But in this case it is not so. The spectrum being of bright lines, the light is localized and readily impresses the plate. Moreover, any error in the rate of the clock or any tremors of the instrument, which are fatal to the nebula, count for little in photographing its spectrum; since the image is thereby simply shifted off the slit and no injury results to the definition. Many excellent photographs of the spectrum of the nebula in Orion were obtained by Dr. Draper, however, the chief interest in which consists in the fact that beside the characteristic bright lines, there are traces of continuous spectrum in various parts of the nebula, suggesting the beginning of condensation.

Beside the work done at his observatory at Hastings, which may be called astronomical work proper, Dr. Draper occupied himself with collateral questions of not less importance, in the admirably equipped physical laboratory he had built in connection with his residence in New York City. It was here, in 1873, that he made the exquisite, and to this day unequaled photograph of the diffraction p=spectrum. The region from wave-length 4850, below G, to wave-length 8440 near O, was contained upon a single plate. The Roman astronomer Secchi reproduced this photograph as a steel plate for his great work on the Sun, and the British Association, in 1880, endorsed it as the best known standard spectrum by publishing a lithograph of it in their Proceedings. The grating used to produce this photograph was one of Mr. Rutherford's superb plates, ruled with 6481 lines to the inch. It was in his New York laboratory, too, that he made the most important discovery of his life, perhaps; that of the existence of oxygen in the sun. After months of laborious and costly experiment, he succeeded, in 1876, in photographing the solar spectrum and the spectrum of an incandescent gas upon the same plate, with their edges in complete contact; thus enabling the coincidence or non-coincidence of the lines in the two spectra to be established beyond a doubt.

On examining the spectrum of oxygen thus photographed, he saw that while the lines of the iron and the aluminum used as electrodes, coincided, as they should do, with their proper dark lines in the sun's spectrum, the lines of oxygen agreed with bright solar lines. Whence the important conclusion announced by him, 1st, that oxygen actually existed in the sun, now for the first time proved; and, 2d, that this gas exists there under conditions either of temperature or pressure, or both, which enable it to radiate more light than the contiguous portions of the solar mass. This view of the case however, required radical modification in the then accepted view of the constitution of the sun; a modification which he pointed out and advocated.

So exceptional were these results, and especially the conclusions from them, that it was hardly to be expected that they should be at once accepted. Dr. Draper, however, in this, as in all his work, was his own severest critic. Increasing constantly his appliances and perfecting his methods he produced, in 1879, another photograph on a much larger scale, which showed the coincidences which he claimed, especially of groups of lines, so unmistakably as to leave no question of the fact in a mind free from bias. To strengthen still more the evidence on the subject, he had planned for the execution the present winter, a research upon the spectra of other non-metallic gases, in the hope that some of these, too, would be found represented as bright lines in the sun spectrum.

In 1878, he was the director of a party organized by himself to observe the total eclipse of the sun of the 29th of July. His familiarity with the locality led him to select Rawlins, Wyoming, an important station on the Union Pacific Railway, as the objective point. The result justified his selection. The expedition was entirely successful, and the observations which were made were of great value. By means of his splendid apparatus, Dr. Draper himself obtained an excellent photograph of the corona and also a photograph of its diffraction spectrum, which was apparently continuous.

In 1880, he obtained a number of spectra of Jupiter in connection with stellar work. On examining one of these spectra, the photograph appeared to him to show that the planet really furnished a certain amount of intrinsic light. The exposure on Jupiter was fifty minutes, the spectrum of the moon being taken in ten. The original negative was sent over to his friend, Mr. A. C. Ranyard, who presented it to the Royal Astronomical Society. In June, 1881, he took several excellent photographs of the comet, and also of its spectrum. With a slit and two prisms he obtained three photographs of the spectrum, with exposures of 180, 196, and 228 minutes, respectively. On each plate, a comparison spectrum was also photographed.

Upon the organization of the United States Commission to observe the Transit of Venus in 1874, Dr. Draper's great attainments in celestial photography pointed him out at once as the man best suited to organize the photographic section, and he was accordingly appointed Director of the Photographic Department. He went at once to Washington, entered heartily into the work, and during three entire months devoted himself to the labor of organizing, experimenting and instructing; declining subsequently all compensation for the time thus spent.

Although his duties at home prevented him from joining any of the expeditions, yet so instrumental had he been in making the transit observations a success, that upon the recommendation of the Commission, Congress ordered a gold medal to be struck in his honor at the Philadelphia Mint. This medal is 46 millimeters in diameter. It has the representation of a siderostat in relief upon the obverse, with the motto: "Famam extendere factis, hoc virtutis opus." On the reverse is inscribed the words: "Veneris in sole spectandae curatores R. P. F. S. Henrico Draper, M. D., Dec. VIII, MDCCCLXXIV;" with this motto: "Decori decus addit avito."

Professor Draper was appointed, in 1861, Surgeon of the Twelfth Regiment of New York Volunteers; a position which he accepted and in which he served with credit. In 1876, he was made one of the Judges in the Photographic Section of the Centennial Exhibition. In 1875, he was elected a member of the Astronomische Gesellschaft. In 1877, he received an election to the National Academy of Sciences; and in the same year he was made a member of the American Philosophical Society. In 1879, he was elected a Fellow of the American Association for the Advancement of Science. In 1881, the American Academy of Arts and Sciences worthily enrolled him among its members. In 1882, the University of Wisconsin and the University of New York conferred on him, almost simultaneously, the degree of LL.D.

For several years it had been Dr. Draper's custom to join his friends, Generals Marcy and Whipple, of the Army, in the early fall, for a few weeks' hunting in the Rocky mountains. In 1882, the party left New York on the 31st of August, went by rail to Rock creek, on the Union Pacific Railway, and from there went north in the saddle; reaching Fort Custer, on the Northern Pacific Railway, near the middle of October. During the two months of their absence the party rode fifteen hundred miles on horseback, as Dr. Draper estimated. When above timber line early in October, they encountered a blinding snow storm with intense cold and were obliged to camp without shelter.

Dr. Draper reached New York on the 25th of October. Ordinarily, he returned refreshed and invigorated with the splendid exercise of the trip; but this year the distance traveled seemed to have been too great, and this, together with the hardships encountered, seemed to have wearied him. Pressure of delayed business awaited him and occupied his time at once. Moreover, the National Academy was to meet in New York in November; and he was to entertain them as he had always done.

This year the entertainment was to take the form of a dinner. In order to offer them scientific novelty, he determined to light the table with the Edison incandescent light, the current being furnished from the machine in his laboratory. But the source of power being a gas engine, and therefore intermittent, a disagreeable pulsation was observable in the light. To obviate this he contrived an ingenious attachment to the engine whereby at the instant at which the speed was accelerated by the explosion of the gas in the cylinder, a lateral or shunt circuit should be automatically thrown in, the resistance of which could be varied at pleasure. With his admirable mechanical skill he extemporized the device from materials at hand and found it to work perfectly.

The dinner was given on the evening of November 15th, and was one of the most brilliant ever given in New York; about forty academicians, together with a few personal friends as invited guests, sitting at table. But Dr. Draper's overwork now told upon him; slightly indisposed as he had been before, he was unable to partake of food, and a premonitory chill seized him while at the table. As soon as the dinner was over, he took a hot bath, thinking thus to throw it off. But while in the bath a second and severe chill of a decidedly congestive type attacked him, and it was only with the greatest difficulty that he could be carried to his bed.

His warm friend and former colleague, Dr. Metcalfe, was at once summoned and pronounced the attack double pleuritis. The best of treatment and the most careful nursing seemed for two or three days to be producing an effect for the better. But on the Sunday following, heart complications developed and he died about 4 o'clock in the morning of Monday, the 20th of November.

Viewed from whatever standpoint, the life of Henry Draper appears as successful as it was earnest, honest and pure. His devotion to science was supreme; to him no labor was too severe, no sacrifice too great, if by it he could approach nearer the exact truth. The researches he had already made, and much more those he had projected, involved the largest expenditure of his time and means. But such was his delight in his scientific work, and his enthusiasm in carrying it on, that he was never happier than when hardest at work in his laboratory, never more cheerful than when most zealously laboring with his superb telescopes.

Moreover, he was as eminent as a teacher of science as he was as an investigator. His lectures were simple, clear and forcible. They held the interest of the class and awakened their enthusiasm while they enriched the student's store of knowledge and strengthened his powers of observation and of reason. In the laboratory he was keen, thorough and impartial, while at the same time considerate and helpful; ever striving to encourage honest endeavor and to assist the earnest worker.

Still another sphere of labor, however, made demands upon his time. In 1867, he married Mary

Anna, the accomplished daughter of Courtlandt Palmer, of New York. Upon Mr. Palmer's death, in 1874, Dr. Draper became the managing trustee of an immense estate and, with his characteristic energy and efficiency, entered at once upon the task of reducing it to a basis of maximum production with the minimum amount of attention. The responsibility which thus rested upon him, the harassing demands of tenants, the endless details of leases, contracts and deeds, and the no less annoying complications of necessary law suits, worried him incessantly. And had it not been for his unsurpassed business capacity, he might have failed. But he was equal to the demand upon him, and within a few years, order had come out of confusion, and a few hours at his office daily enabled all to flow along smoothly.

To indicate the esteem in which Dr. Draper was held by his confreres in science, the following passages may be quoted from an excellent biographical notice of him written by Professor Young, of Princeton: "In person he was of medium height, compactly built, with a pleasing address, and a keen black eye which missed nothing within its range. He was affectionate, noble, just and generous; a thorough gentleman, with a quick and burning contempt for all shame and meanness; a friend most kind, sympathetic, helpful, and brotherly, genial, wise and witty in conversation; clear-headed, prudent and active in business; a man of the highest and most refined intellectual tastes and qualities; a lover of art and music, and also of manly sports, especially the hunt; of such manual skill that no mechanic in the city could do finer work than he; in the pursuit of science, able, indefatigable, indomitable, sparing neither time, labor nor expense."

"Excepting his early death, Dr. Draper was a man fortunate in all things; in his vigorous physique, his delicate senses, and skillful hand; in his birth and education; in his friendships; and especially in his marriage, which brought to him not only wealth and all the happiness which naturally comes with a lovely, true-hearted and faithful wife, but also a most unusual companionship and intellectual sympathy in all his favorite pursuits. He was fortunate in the great resources which lay at his disposal, and in the wisdom to manage and use them well; in the subjects he chose for his researches and in the complete success he invariably attained."

Such a man as this it is whose name we are sorrowfully called upon to strike from the roll of our living membership. Professor Draper was a man among men, a scientist of the highest type. Stricken down in the midst of his life work, at the early age of 45, the bright promise of his noble life is left unfulfilled. What brilliant researches in his favorite science he would have made, we can never know. But with a mind so richly endowed and so thoroughly trained, with an experimental ability as earnest as it was persistent, with facilities for investigation which were as perfect as they are rare, with abundance of time and means at his disposal, and above all, with a devoted wife, who keenly appreciated the value of his scientific work, was ever at his side as his trusty assistant and always shared in the glory and the honor of his discoveries, we may be sure that, had he been permitted to reach the age of his honored father, results would have been reaped by his labors which would have added still brighter lustre to the science of America.

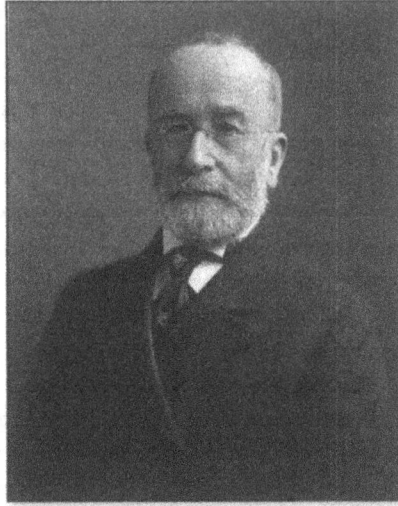

WILLIAM WILLIAMS KEEN

1837–1932 (APS 1884)

Memoir by William Darrach

Our Society has never left its members nor the public in doubt as to its function. This is stated in its full name—The American Philosophical Society, for the Promotion of Useful Knowledge. Promotion—moving forward—upward—the word not only suggests progress—motion forward, but also to a higher plane.

Knowledge can be promoted in many ways. In the lead we find the pioneer investigators, who, by their mental processes and experiments create new knowledge, ascertain new facts, establish new principles, open up new vistas of thought and action. Then, there are those who apply these new ideas and principles to facts already known and perfect the technique of their usefulness. Knowledge is also promoted by those who having learned by themselves, or from others, teach this knowledge—the spreaders of the gospel. They teach their own confreres and their younger students and the public at large. They teach by their writings, by word of mouth, in lectures and in conversation. They also teach by their examples.

But to be a pioneer, or a teacher or both, one must be ever a student. To be any of these, one must have an unappeasable hunger. One must desire to learn new truths and one must desire to help others to learn. The true teacher must do more than impart information to his listener; he must create in him that same hunger to acquire knowledge; he must stimulate him to think for himself until he too becomes a creator of new and useful knowledge. The true teacher should be to those who work with him, what water is to the desert as it flows through the irrigating ditch to transform the barren land from a gray, sterile, inactive bit of the earth's surface, to something green and alive and productive.

It is from this point of view that I ask you to consider with me one whom recent memory will call to mind as a little old man, quite frail and somewhat tottery, but still full of that marvelous optimism and cheer and human interest that lasted so vitally over a long stretch of years. William Williams Keen was a promoter of useful knowledge. He was a pioneer in his chosen fields of both anatomy and surgery. By experiment and by investigation he brought to light new facts and new principles. This new knowledge as well as that he learned from others, he applied to the art of surgery.

In 1876 he heard Lister describe the principles of antiseptic surgery and became so convinced of their truth that he applied them at once at St. Mary's Hospital. He was one of the earliest American surgeons to adopt this all important advance in surgery. He continued to develop its technique until it merged into the aseptic surgery of later days. His courageous pioneer work in the surgery of the brain was not reckless plunging into unknown territory, but was based on sound training, first as a young co-worker with Weir Mitchell, secondly as head of the old Philadelphia School of Anatomy, and thirdly when, as editor of a new edition of Gray's Anatomy, he had to rewrite the chapter on the brain. So, as opportunities for cerebral surgery came, they found him well prepared to undertake them wisely.

The association with Weir Mitchell was one of the most treasured incidents of his career, as he was proud to testify on many occasions. He said "his was the most stimulating mind I have ever been in contact with." In 1863, Mitchell requested Surgeon General Hammond to transfer Keen to the hospital where he and Morehouse were already installed. Years later, Mitchell told him the reason for this request was that he had already found that he could never kill him with hard work.

This tireless energy was perhaps the dominant characteristic of the man both mentally and physically. Soon after he arrived at Brown University in 1854 he realized that his school preparation had been inferior to that of many of his classmates. His reaction to this was redoubled effort and as a result he graduated at the head of his class. The subject of his valedictory address was "The Scholar's Sentiment of Veneration for the Past." Five years earlier, on graduating from high school, his essay was "The Prospect of Man." One may say that these topics illustrate his courage.

It is worthy of note that having chosen medicine as his career he decided to spend an additional year of preparation at Brown. Thorough premedical education was rather rare in those days. His mornings were spent in chemistry and physics and the afternoons in English literature. The results of this latter effort can be seen in his clear, forceful style both in lectures and writings and in his careful work as editor.

We next find him at Jefferson and in the offices of Jacob Da Costa and John Brinton. Between the two sessions he was Assistant Surgeon in the Army and was active in the first Battle of Bull Run. After receiving his medical degree in March, 1862, he reentered the army and served until 1864, the latter part of this period being with Weir Mitchell and Morehouse at the special nerve hospital on Christian Street. His army career was then interrupted for 53 years but in 1917 we find him a Major in the Medical Corps, serving on the Medical Council.

After the Civil War there followed a period of study abroad, in Berlin with Virchow and later in Paris. In 1866 he returned to Philadelphia and began his long career of teaching and practice. He almost immediately took over the Philadelphia School of Anatomy, that extramural institution which had been founded in 1820 by Lawrance, in which Godman, Pancoast and Agnew had preceded him. In addition, he was appointed to teach surgical pathology at Jefferson. When Joseph Pancoast resigned from the Chair of Anatomy in 1873, Keen tried hard for the appointment, but without success

Defeat only spurred him to greater efforts and he became more occupied with his surgical work. In 1884, he was appointed Professor of Surgery in the Woman's Medical College, which position he held for five years. During this period he began his work in cerebral surgery and at the First Congress of American Physicians and Surgeons in Washington in 1888 he presented three patients from whom he had removed brain tumors.

In his 53rd year, he was appointed Professor of Surgery in the Jefferson Medical College, succeeding the younger Gross. As he says "it was very late to begin a career" but for the next eighteen years he was most active as a surgeon, as a teacher and as a writer. In 1907 he resigned his professorship and retired from surgical practice, clinching the latter by eighteen months of travel abroad.

On his return home, he immediately resumed his energetic career. He had given up the scalpel but only to replace it with a pen. In 1905 he had commenced work on his System of Surgery. The last of eight volumes was brought out in 1921, each one containing about 1,000 pages. It contains articles by 138 different American and British authors. Each of these was planned and carefully edited by Keen himself, some being largely rewritten. In 1908 he began a ten year service as President of this Society. His interest in his Alma Mater was always active and he served as Trustee of Brown University from 1873 until his death.

Few men have championed the cause of animal experimentation more forcefully or actively than he did, beginning with a Commencement address at the Woman's Medical College in 1885, and continuing until almost the end of his days.

He was a deeply religious man and an active member and supporter of the Baptist church.

His list of honors included many degrees and positions of distinction both at home and abroad. As he himself wrote "Both my professional and other friends have literally showered honors upon me, far more than I have ever deserved. I say this advisedly, for I think I appraise my abilities and my services far more clearly and exactly than these, my over generous friends, have done."

He was particularly proud of being elected President of the International Surgical Association in 1914. Because of the war, the next meeting was not held until 1920. At the age of 83 he not only went to Paris to preside but spent a good deal of the preceding months in studying French so that he might better use the language of the hosts of the Society.

His complete bibliography fills many pages of titles of books and papers on anatomy, surgery — both civil and military, and on immortality. Through these writings he was most active and efficient as a spreader of the gospel. During his long period as a teacher, he was himself what he called Mitchell, a "yeasty man." He fermented others. Even after his retirement, he continued to impart information and to stimulate others to think.

He was a brilliant conversationalist and a most active correspondent. I know of one dean of a medical school in another city who looked forward to the monthly letter from Spruce Street. Each one meant not only an answer but a definite chore to be done, but one always worth doing. It was hard to resist that glowing enthusiasm, that young point of view, that eager optimism, that catholic, broad outlook. Nor could one easily fail to be infected by those merry twinkling eyes and the ready laugh.

He was a clean man who hated vulgarity. He was a loyal man, loyal to the ideals of his profession, loyal to his friends. He was always interested in young men, stimulating them, ready to listen to their theories, believing in them. His triumphant, firm belief in immortality was an outstanding quality. Few men have been members of this Society for 48 years and fewer yet have as consistently carried out its function of promoting useful knowledge. For more than ninety years he was a grand, young man!

EDITORS' NOTE

During much of his long life of 99 years the colorful W. W. Keen was arguably the nation's or even the world's most famous surgeon. During the Civil War he served as an Army surgeon even before he finished medical school. After completing medical school and surgical training he became the first to successfully remove a brain tumor and one of the first in America to adopt Lister's antiseptic surgical technique. He was President of the International Surgical Society, the AMA and the APS. Surprisingly the most famous episode in W. W. Keen's life is not mentioned in Dr. Darrach's memoir. Perhaps he assumed it was so well known to APS members that he needn't include it. This was Dr. Keen's participation in a clandestine operation on President Grover Cleveland. The reason for secrecy was that during the country's financial crisis of 1893 the President was diagnosed with a malignant tumor in his mouth. The country's financial turmoil had been caused by Congress passing the inflationary Sherman Silver Purchase Act which threatened to undermine the US Treasury's gold reserve. Cleveland's leadership appeared essential for repeal of the Act. It was thought that if the story got out that the President had cancer and might soon be disabled, the country would plunge further into financial panic. Therefore a covert operation was planned for removal of the tumor. This was conducted on a private yacht as it steamed up Long Island Sound ostensibly carrying a perfectly healthy President Cleveland to his vacation. Dr. Joseph Bryant of New York and W. W. Keen were the surgeons. Resection of the tumor required removal of a large portion of the patient's upper jaw. Amazingly Bryant and Keen managed to accomplish this without any external incisions by working entirely within the mouth. They then replaced the President's palate with a prosthesis thus enabling him to speak normally only days later at a special session of Congress. As a result the Sherman Act was repealed, the Nation's financial panic was avoided and for another 15 years the President survived. For 24 years all this was kept secret until Keen reported it in a 1917 article in the Saturday Evening Post.

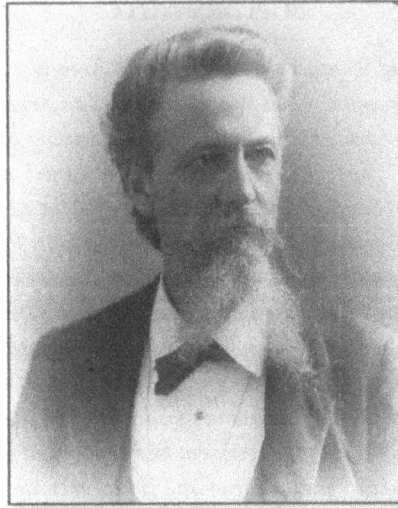

WILLIAM GIBSON ARLINGTON BONWILL

1833–1899 (APS 1885)

Memoir by C. Newlin Peirce

He was elected a member of the American Philosophical Society October 16, 1885. He was the oldest son and second child of Dr. William Moore Bonwill and Louisa Mason Baggs, his wife.

Dr. William Moore Bonwill was born in Delaware, but his father was of English parentage. He first settled in Canterbury, Del., but soon removed to Camden, Del., where he practiced medicine for forty years. Both the father and grandfather of the subject of this biography were noted for natural ability and genius in mechanics, and it was this gift which was of such service to both father and son, one in the practice of general surgery, and the other in that of dental surgery.

Dr. W. G. A. Bonwill, from his seventh to his fourteenth year, attended school in the academy of Middletown, Del., where his course of instruction included algebra, geometry, chemistry and some elementary Latin and Greek.

Leaving school at an early age, he was thrown upon his own resources, and accepted any honest employment he could find. It was with much pride and pleasure that he narrated his experience as carpenter, cabinet maker, clerk in store and school teacher, until finally the dental laboratory of Dr. Samuel W. Neall, of Camden, N. J., became the scene of his activity for six months. This brief apprenticeship was, however, supplemented by three months spent with two of Baltimore's most prominent dentists, Drs. Chapin A. Harris and A. A. Blandy.

In October, 1854, Dr. Bonwill commenced the practice of dentistry in Dover, Del. His previous experience in the mechanical industries was now of great service to him, enabling him with little expense to make all the necessary appurtenances of his office and laboratory. Thus, as he was proud to narrate, "with one suit of clothes and $3 in my pocket," he entered upon a professional career in which he won the admiration and confidence of his associates, and a competency for himself and family.

In 1866 he graduated from the Pennsylvania College of Dental Surgery, and subsequently received the degree of M.D. from the Jefferson Medical College. In 1871 he removed to Philadelphia, believing that the larger city would offer better opportunities for his advancement. He lived abstemiously, especially as to his diet, so that his energy and persistence served him throughout his career. His motto was always to finish every day the matter in hand. This habit enabled him to accomplish much laborious work.

Besides the numerous dental societies of which he was either an active or an honorary member in the United States and foreign countries, he was a member of the Union League, the Art Club, The Historical Society, and The Academy of Natural Sciences. While his talent was appreciated at home, his reputation was probably greater abroad. He was an honorary member of Russian, Dutch, German, Spanish and French dental societies, from each of which he received decorations and honors; and by the Franklin Institute of Philadelphia he was awarded the Cresson gold medal for his invention of the Electro-Magnetic Mallet, which was patented by him in 1878

His first Dental Engine was patented in 1874; in 1876 his invention of the Diamond Reamer was announced, a rapidly revolving diamond point, the use of which was for permanently destroying contact of approximating surfaces of the teeth. But while efficient for the purpose intended, his own modification of methods in practice soon withdrew it from the profession.

His Cord Dental Engine, popularly known as the Bonwill Dental Engine, which embodied the essential principles of the Bonwill Surgical Engine, was patented in 1877. In this instrument he took great pride, especially so in consequence of its service to the general surgeon, claiming that this engine stands as an evidence of how much can be accomplished in surgery by machinery.

His manipulative skill made him a remarkably popular clinical teacher. He made numerous operations in gold which were elaborate and wonderful, while in his use of plastics, especially amalgam, no one could excel him in beautiful and exact restorations.

As a teacher he was interesting, instructive and novel, his method was his own—he gave freely to all who desired. He had implicit faith in his own ideas—his ambition was to make them known and so perpetuate them. A fertile writer, though often presenting his thoughts in such form that the kernel of truth was not grasped, unless the readers were willing to delve beneath the externals by subsequent conferences with the author.

His most important papers were as follows: "The Electro-Magnetic Mallet," in 1874; "The Air an Anesthetic," 1878; "The Salvation of the Human Teeth," 1881; "Plastic Gold Alloys," 1882; "Geometrical and Mechanical Laws of Articulation," 1885; "Regulators and Methods of Correcting Irregularities," 1887; "New Method of Clasped Plates vs. Bridge Work," 1890; "What Has Dentistry to Demonstrate Against the Hypothesis of Organic Evolution?" 1893.

Dr. Bonwill was a genius. In common with others thus peculiarly organized, he had a wonderful facility for misinterpreting the acts of others, believing himself persecuted, while there was no real reason for grief or offense. The reception with which his essay of 1893, "Demonstration Against the Hypothesis of Organic Evolution," met among his warmest friends was a source of great disappointment and discomfort. His ambition and his appreciation of himself as a scientific observer were wounded, for he had great faith that the principles therein enunciated would not only check the acceptance of this, as he believed, false theory, but would reestablish the ancient doctrine of special creations.

The profession Dr. Bonwill loved, and for and in which he labored, has profited by his genius more than is now realized. With his demise disappears a unique and forceful personality—one of the most conspicuous and remarkable characters ever associated with the profession of dentistry.

He cannot be judged by the standard of ordinary men, for he was not ordinary, either in thought or action. Naturally versatile, his many-sided character presented itself to his associates in such manner as to lead to varied estimates of him. In temperament, nervously active, he was not content to labor as others—his whole energy was concentrated upon whatever for the time being occupied him. Aggressive and fearless, criticism was to him a stimulant to renewed activity, and, as he often stated, failure did not enter his mind as a possibility.

With the temperament of an artist and the talent of a mechanician, he had a lively imagination and a love of the beautiful. These qualities, added to his intense activity, made him fertile in inventions which are connected with his name, and which have made him, in dentistry, well known throughout the world. He made mistakes, but he did not hesitate to acknowledge them upon conclusive evidence of his error. Generous in his impulses, but erratic in his attachment to his friends, those who knew him best will most regret his absence, and many to him unknown, to whom his life had been helpful, will feel that the fullness and ripeness of his years have been prematurely curtailed.

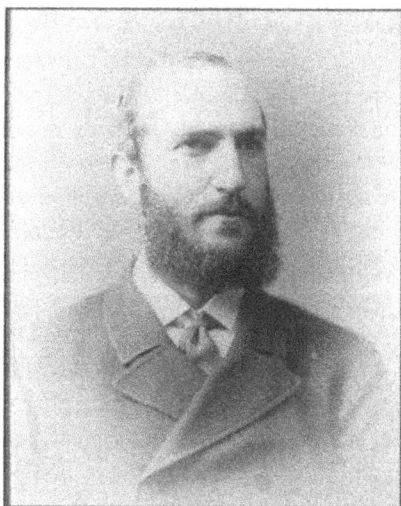

I. MINIS HAYS

1847–1925 (APS 1886)

Memoir by APS Library staff

Isaac Minis Hays was a Philadelphia physician, ophthalmologist, editor and librarian. He was the editor of the American Journal of the Medical Sciences from 1878–1890. He later became Secretary and Librarian of the American Philosophical Society from 1897–1922. As APS Librarian, he collected and cataloged the great mass of Benjamin Franklin's papers for the American Philosophical Society. He also published a Calendar of Franklin Papers (1907) and a Chronology of Benjamin Franklin (2nd ed., 1913).

Hays was born in Philadelphia on July 26, 1847, the son of Dr. Isaac Hays (1796–1879, APS 1863) and Sarah Minis. He was sent to the Classical Institute for his secondary education, and afterward matriculated at the University of Pennsylvania. He graduated A.B. in 1866 and immediately entered Penn's medical school, graduating M.D. in 1868. Remaining an extra year, he took a Master of Arts degree in 1869. Also, in 1869 he became the assistant editor to his father Isaac Hays, who was the editor of the American Journal of Medical Sciences.

Hays wrote or edited several works in his field of ophthalmology, including the American edition of J. Soelberg Wells's *Treatise on the Diseases of the Eye* (1873) and a statistical survey, entitled "Blindness: Its Frequency, Causes and Prevention" for William F. Norris and Charles A. Oliver's *System of Diseases of the Eye* (1897). However, Hays took little pleasure in the practice of medicine (having few patients) or in medical research.

Hays succeeded his father as editor of the *American Journal of Medical Sciences*, after his father's death in 1878. Already as assistant editor, he had commissioned four historical articles to demonstrate American contributions over the previous century to Medicine, Surgery, Obstetrics and Gynecology.

133

These appeared in successive quarterly issues of the *Journal* in 1876, and were reprinted as a monograph entitled, *A Century of American Medicine*. Several years after becoming editor, Hays converted a sister publication of the *Journal*, the monthly *Medical News and Library*, to a weekly format. He conceived the publication, containing extracts from other journals, as a "medium" for "transmitting the earliest intelligence of medical discoveries and progress," and recruited special correspondents in other cities for this purpose. These endeavors gave Hays a notable reputation as a medical editor.

Hays's earliest experiences with libraries came after his election as a Fellow of the College of Physicians of Philadelphia in 1872. The following year he was appointed to the Library Committee of the College, and pursued its work with creativity and energy. One of his greatest concerns was to see that the College library was properly cataloged, and he visited the Library Company of Philadelphia and the Boston Medical Library to learn about the costs, materials and systems for cataloging the collection. He even concerned himself with the particulars of the library's operations, designing charge slips, helping to draft rules for the use of the library, drafting a new, expanded schedule for its hours of operation, binding library and archival materials and hiring its first professional staff. As the College Librarian became more experienced in his post, the need for the Library Committee to be involved in the day-to-day operations lessened. Hays was displeased by this "restriction" in the Committee's authority, and offered his resignation in 1893.

Hays' earlier editorial and library committee assignments would be excellent preparation for his work at the American Philosophical Society. He was elected to membership in the Society in February of 1886, and eleven years later became one of its secretaries. He was also appointed acting librarian to replace of Dr. George H. Horn (1840–1897, APS 1869), who had fallen ill. Within a few weeks of his new appointments he began initiatives for changes that would occupy the Society for a quarter of a century. Serving as the APS Librarian, secretary and editor, Hays was effectively its first executive officer. During the twenty-five year period from 1897–1922 he is said to have written 48,000 letters on Society business and edited twenty-seven volumes of the *Proceedings* and *Transactions*. With a passion for order, a keen analytical sense, and abundant physical energy, he became the driving force behind all of the Society's work.

Drawing upon his experiences on the Library Committee of the College of Physicians, Hays brought needed changes to the Society's Library. On his appointment as Acting Librarian, he was invited to sit on the Library Committee and began making important recommendations. Later, after the death of the former Librarian Dr. Horn in 1898, Hays became an ex officio member of the Library Committee. Among his first recommendations were the establishment of rules governing the operation of the Library, the purchase of a card catalog, and the hiring of a professional cataloger. Other library staff was added over the next few years, totaling four by 1901. For a library cataloging system Hays adopted the Dewey Decimal Classification system to replace the "philosophical" classification of former APS Librarian J. Peter Lesley (1819–1903, APS 1856). Next, he turned to the Library's neglected books and periodicals that were badly in need of binding. He identified and sold duplicate volumes and withdrew books outside the Library's fields of interest, donating many pamphlets on Unitarian theology (garnered by the Society's first Librarian John Vaughan (1756–1841, APS 1784) to the First Unitarian Church. Hays extended the hours during which the Library was open to readers, and also asked for increased space. One of his most impressive accomplishments was a fifteen-year project to bind and catalog the papers of Benjamin Franklin.

Having proceeded with the organization of the Library, Hays now turned to the APS Committee on Historical Manuscripts for advice about how to make the Society's many large collections accessible to researchers. On the Committee's recommendation calendars were prepared for the papers of Richard Henry Lee, Nathanael Greene and General George Weedon. Hays is best known outside the Society for promoting the Benjamin Franklin papers, donated to the Society by Charles Pemberton Fox in 1840. This collection was little known or used for much of the nineteenth century, although Paul L. Ford used it extensively for his 1899 portrait, *The Many-Sided Franklin*.

Shortly after Hays' appointment as Librarian, APS member Talcott Williams (1849–1928, APS 1888) suggested to him that a calendar be prepared for the Franklin papers. Hays presented the idea of a Franklin Collection calendar to the APS Council along with a proposal that the Society celebrate the bicentennial of Franklin's birth in 1906. Neither proposal was adopted. Consequently, he changed his tactics. In the final paper of a scientific session at the General Meeting that year, the Chairman of the Library Committee Joseph G. Rosengarten (1835–1921, APS 1891) described the content and character of the Franklin papers, expressing the hope that a calendar might be prepared for the collection in the not too distant future— "certainly by the two hundredth anniversary of the birth of our founder." In the business meeting that followed Hays gained unanimous consent for a committee "to prepare a plan for the appropriate celebration of the bicentennial of the birth of Franklin."

The plans for a bicentennial celebration of Franklin's birth drew widespread support, from the U.S. government, the Pennsylvania legislature, and the city of Philadelphia. On April 20, 1906 dignitaries from across the nation and the globe assembled in Philadelphia to celebrate the bicentennial. These included Senator Henry Cabot Lodge, leading the congressional delegation; Ambassador Jean A.A. J. Jusserand (1855–1932, APS 1907), representing the French Republic; as well as delegates from 127 learned societies. In addition to addresses on Franklin by leading scholars, there were luncheons, dinners and two academic convocations. There were also memorial ceremonies at Franklin's grave. The grateful members of the Society recognized Hays' achievement with an illuminated scroll and an engraved silver cup. After the departure of guests, the Committee on the Franklin Bicentennial directed Hays to prepare a memorial volume and "to secure the services of a corps of assistants to complete the Calendar of the Franklin papers." The calendar appeared in five large volumes in 1908.

As APS Secretary Hays resuscitated the spirit of the Society just as he had revived its Library. By the last decade of the nineteenth century, attendance at the Society's semi-monthly meetings was meager. The number of attendees rarely reached thirty. In 1901 Hays proposed that the Society hold an annual general meeting, lasting several days to attract distant members instead of the semi-monthly meetings. His plan was approved, and the first general meeting was held on April 3–5, 1902 and was a resounding success. 115 members attended, and such meetings became a regular feature of the Society's calendar. Sometimes the general meetings were planned around an anniversary or special theme like the centennial of Darwin's birth. In 1910 ordinary meetings were reduced to one a month, and in 1936 monthly meetings were dropped completely in favor of a second general meeting.

Hays' other major initiative within the American Philosophical Society was less successful. The reawakening of the members' interest in the Society and its mission naturally produced a desire for larger quarters. This was especially the case, since member attendance at general meetings had grown significantly and the library had outstripped the available space. As a matter of fact, in 1912 some books from the Library's collection had to be put into storage at a neighboring bank. At this time in Philadelphia the new Parkway was taking shape under the leadership of former Fairmount Park Commissioner Eli Kirk Price, Jr. (1860–1933, APS 1916), who based the plans upon the model of the Champs d' Elysees in Paris. Hays was among the Society's members, who voted to leave the Philosophical Hall facility on Independence Square and to construct a new building at 16th and Cherry streets. To this end he mounted a fund-raising campaign, playing a large part in the related meetings, discussions and publicity. However, the advent of World War I diverted the attention of the members and the public for a number of years. In 1922 before the relocation scheme could be realized, the city of Philadelphia decided to use the 16th and Cherry Street tract for a park.

In the spring of 1922 Hays shocked the members of the American Philosophical Society with an announcement of his retirement. The members were genuinely dismayed, since few active members could recall a time when he had not been in charge. After his resignation, Hays continued to be an active and outspoken APS member. Among his activities, he was appointed Chairman of the Committee on Library, and in this capacity he wrote an article on Benjamin Franklin's Canada pamphlet entitled, *The Interest of Great Britain Considered* (1760), as well as answering questions from a new generation of Franklin scholars such as George Simpson Eddy. In 1924 Hays served as secretary of a special committee to plan an international scientific conference to celebrate the Society's two hundredth anniversary in 1926. He presented his plan for the celebration on May 27, 1925. Unfortunately, he would not live to see it realized. Ten days later, the seventy-seven year old Hays died of a heart attack on June 5, during a heat wave of unseasonable intensity. In his will Hays directed that after the death of his daughters, the income of his considerable estate should be paid to the American Philosophical Society, the institution he had served for thirty-seven years.

EDITORS' NOTE

The name I. Minis Hays should be familiar to APS members since the following passage appears in the program for each meeting. "On this occasion, we gratefully remember the services to the Society of I. Minis Hays, Secretary and Librarian, 1897-1922, whose generous bequest included a modest sum for entertainment at our stated Meetings."

In his will, Dr. Hays specified that his bequest "for entertainment" should continue to be acknowledged in perpetuity. If it was not the trust fund he established for the APS was to be transferred to the Library Company. Compliance with his wish is worth our attention. The "modest sum" helps to pay for the members' lunch at each annual meeting. In addition since Dr. Hays' Trust has appreciated and now totals over $4 million. What's left of the income after paying for lunch is very useful in supporting the library.

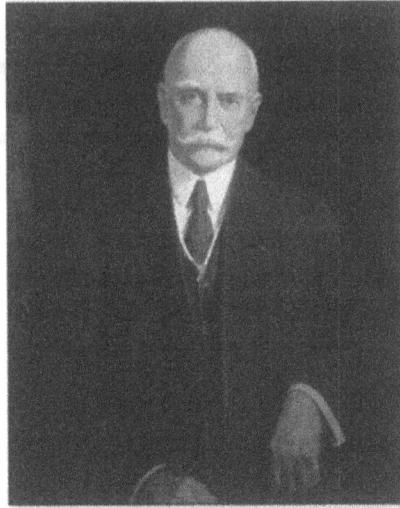

FRANCIS X. DERCUM

1856–1931 (APS 1892)

Memoir by Albert P. Brubaker

Dr. Francis X. Dercum, the late President of the American Philosophical Society was a distinguished physician and neurologist of Philadelphia and highly esteemed and honored by his colleagues at home and abroad. He was also a student of Biology and deeply interested in many of its problems partly for their intrinsic value and partly for the light thrown, by their solution, on the phenomena of the human body both in health and disease. Neurology and biology were his two major interests.

Dr. Francis X. Dercum, a native of Philadelphia was born August 10, 1856. He was the son of Ernest Albert and Susanna Erhart Dercum. He was a descendant of a line of European ancestors many of whom were distinguished as lawyers, judges, scholars, scientists and physicians. Two of these ancestors occupied professorial chairs in the University of Wurzburg in Germany. It might be expected coming from such an ancestry that he would inherit some of the traits that characterized and distinguished his predecessors "His forebears of old."

Dr. Dercum's grandfather and father came from Germany. They immigrated to this country in consequence of the failure of the revolutionary movement in 1848 to obtain a more liberalized form of government and with the leaders of which they had been sympathetically allied. Dr. Dercum's early education was received primarily in the public schools of Philadelphia and secondarily in the Central High School, the foster mother of many of the distinguished professional men of this City. From this institution he was graduated in 1873, and which later conferred upon him the degree of M.A.

In obedience very probably to an inherited instinct he resolved to study medicine and with this end in view he entered the Medical Department of the University of Pennsylvania in 1874 and from which he was graduated in 1877.

So zealous and assiduous was the young student in the acquisition of knowledge that the University conferred upon him the degree of Ph.D., after an intensive study of the Sciences in the postgraduate summer school. After his graduation he opened an office thinking himself in all probability prepared to engage in the practice of medicine. While waiting for patients which proverbially are slow to appreciate the merits and qualifications of a recent graduate, his mind reverted to the instruction of his university professors especially to that great human and comparative anatomist Dr. Joseph Leidy, who impressed upon him not only a knowledge of the anatomy of the human body but a corresponding knowledge of the anatomy of typical forms of the vertebrate series of animals. From Professor Leidy he received not only that wide view of the unity of organizations of vertebrate animals disclosed by a comparison of their structure, their similarities and dissimilarities but also a love for the biological sciences and an appreciation of the value of the comparative method in the study of the nervous system more especially.

This method was of inestimable service to Dr. Dercum in the years that were to follow. While waiting for patients, Dr. Dercum had many opportunities for reflecting over the problems of comparative anatomy. As a result he prepared two papers, one entitled "On the Sensory Organs, Suggestions with a View to Generalizations"; the other, entitled, "The Morphology of the Semicircular Canals," both of which were published in The American Naturalist, the first in 1878, the second in 1879.

In 1878 Dr. Dercum was elected a member of the Academy of Natural Sciences where he established personal relationships with Leidy, Cope, Ryder, Parker, Chapman and many others by whom his scientific inclinations were strengthened and developed. In the first year of his membership he prepared and read a paper entitled "The Morphology of the Lateral Lines in Fishes," which was subsequently published in the Proceedings of the Academy in 1881.

It was at this time that he made the acquaintance of that gifted and promising anatomist Dr. Andrew J. Parker who was devoting himself to the study of the morphology of the brain with especial reference to the cerebral convolutions not only of man but of the anthropoid apes as well. This subject was attracting the attention of anatomists almost everywhere for the reason that experimental physiologists and clinicians had apparently demonstrated an intimate physical and functional connection between groups of nerve cells of the cerebral cortex and the skeletal muscles on the one hand, and between the sense organs and specialized groups of nerve cells of the cortex on the other hand. As stimulation of the former groups gave rise to muscle movements, and destruction by experimental procedures or disease was followed by a loss of movement or paralysis, they were termed motor centers. As stimulation of the latter group by way of their related sense organs gave rise to sensations, and their destruction by experimental procedures or disease was followed by a loss of sensations peculiar to the sense organs they were termed sensor centers. Both groups of cells came to be regarded as the physical bases of motor and sensor functions.

The bearing of these facts on normal and abnormal conditions of the entire nervous system and its associated organs at once became apparent. Hence it was that the study of the convolutions, their general form, their relations and microscopic structure enlisted the attention and interest of anatomists and neurologists wherever these sciences were cultivated. The friendship of these two young men, which lasted until the untimely death of Dr. Parker, and their mutual interests in the study of the brain, awakened in Dr. Dercum so deep an interest in neurological science that Horatio C. Wood, Professor of Nervous and Mental Diseases in the University of Pennsylvania urged him to devote himself to the study of the diseases of the nervous system. This good suggestion was promptly accepted and conscientiously followed. He was at once in 1883 appointed Chief of the dispensary for nervous diseases, and instructor of nervous diseases in the Medical School of the University, two positions which he held for almost ten years.

With the acceptance of these positions his strictly scientific investigations terminated. In 1887 Dr. Dercum was appointed Neurologist to the Philadelphia Hospital, a position he occupied for 20 years. The dispensary service of the Medical School and the neurological wards of the Philadelphia Hospital were rich in patients who collectively presented so many forms of nervous diseases, that the time and energy of Dr. Dercum were almost wholly occupied with their study and treatment.

Under the stimulating influence and example of Professor H. C. Wood, his interest in and enthusiasm for both nervous and mental diseases increased with his years and as a result he acquired that profound knowledge of his specialty that distinguished him in his subsequent career. Clinical investigations and diagnostic ability were supplemented by a strictly scientific study of the anatomy and physiology of the nervous system both in health and disease.

In 1884 Dr. Dercum in association with Drs. Charles K. Mills, Wharton Sinkler, J. T. Eskridge and others, realized that the relatively new Science of Neurology would be advanced if the neurological students of Philadelphia were given the opportunity to cooperate both in investigations and discussions. For this purpose the Philadelphia Neurological Society was organized, a Society which has had a distinguished career for now forty-seven years. At the meetings of this Society Dr. Dercum presented from time to time a series of papers which enlisted the interest and attention of its members. As a member and subsequently as President, he contributed to the success of its ideals.

During the ten years of his activity in these institutions his alert and active mind observed a great variety of new and strange facts presented by patients with abnormal conditions of the nervous system and the body in general. These facts carefully observed and analyzed formed the subject matter of thirty or more papers written alone or in conjunction with colleagues and which were subsequently published in various medical journals of a general or special character. These contributions to neurological science embraced a wide range of topics, the mere enumeration of which would be out of place in a Memoir of this character especially as their titles are for the most part of a strictly technical character. That they were of sufficient merit to attract the attention of the leading neurologists of the country is apparent from the fact of his admission in 1886 to membership in the American Neurological Association. His interest in the work of this association and his contributions to its annual meetings were highly appreciated, and were rewarded by his associates who elected him Vice-president in 1894-1895, President in 1896 and Councillor in 1897, 1899 and 1905.

In 1892 the Jefferson Medical College created a chair of Nervous and Mental Diseases to which Dr. Dercum was appointed with a seat in the Faculty. This position involved not only the delivery of a systematic course of lectures throughout the academic year but a series of clinical lectures, illustrated by well-selected cases provided by the large and well-organized dispensary service which he founded and developed. In this work he was aided by a large and loyal staff of assistants who contributed in various ways to make the department of nervous and mental diseases a distinguishing feature of the educational work of the Jefferson Medical College.

In this field of professional activity Professor Dercum served the Jefferson Medical College with great distinction for a period of thirty-three years, when he tendered his resignation in the Spring of 1925 much to the regret of the Trustees, the faculty and the student body. Having completed a long. honorable and successful career, he was honored with the unofficial title, Emeritus Professor, which he retained until the day of his death. As a lecturer and teacher, Professor Dercum developed an art of presentation the result of an accurate knowledge of his subject which made him acceptable and instructive to students. His lucidity of statement, his enthusiastic and pleasing delivery won for him unlimited success. The class of 1911 placed on record the general opinion of the student-body in the following words, "Frankness, friendliness, and kindly recognition of the difficulties of his subject and his endeavor to render it less arduous have won for him a place in the heart of every student who has been so fortunate as to come under his tutelage."

By virtue of his knowledge, his acute and logical mind Dr. Dercum was called upon on numerous occasions to testify in the courts of Philadelphia and elsewhere in medico-legal cases in which questions of insanity and other forms of nervous disease were to be considered and judicially decided. So reliable and accurate were his analyses and decisions that he enjoyed for many years an enviable reputation as an expert witness.

The same qualities of mind enabled him to unravel the complex phenomena frequently presented by organic diseases of the nervous system and to determine the location and actual condition of the structures involved. For this reason Dr. Dercum's services as a consultant were much sought after by his professional friends. It was in the capacity of a diagnostic expert that he was called upon from time to time by the neurologists attending President Woodrow Wilson in his long and fatal illness.

Notwithstanding the ever increasing cares and responsibilities of his steadily developing private practice and consultation work, Professor Dercum found time to contribute to neurological science the results of his observations and investigations of nervous and mental diseases. His assiduity in literary work was truly remarkable. The record of his published papers alone during the years from 1892 to 1919 numbers approximately one hundred and seventy titles.

One of the most significant of these papers, published in 1902, was a description of a disorder of nutrition which attracted and still attracts the attention of neurologists. Though some of the individual features of this disorder had doubtless been seen by other clinicians their significance had not been appreciated. It remained for Dr. Dercum to collate and group all the observed features as presented by different patients, to point out their relation one to another and thus give to the groups a distinct entity.

The chief features of this nutritional disorder are large irregular cushion-like deposits of fat in different regions of the body which are painful on pressure, and associated with muscular weakness, ready exhaustion and certain psychic phenomena, as depression, slowness, neurasthenia, hysteria, etc.; to this combination of symptoms Dr. Dercum gave the name Adiposis dolorosa. Subsequently French writers gave to the disease, in honor of its discoverer the name "Maladie de Dercum"—in English speaking countries it is generally referred to as Dercum's disease. The causation has been attributed in recent years to disorders of endocrine organs, more especially to the pituitary.

In the course of his professional life Dr. Dercum was highly honored for his character and achievements by his colleagues at home and in foreign countries. Thus he was elected a member of the Academy of Natural Sciences of Philadelphia in 1878; Fellow of the College of Physicians of Philadelphia in 1885; member of the American Philosophical Society in 1892; President of the American Neurological Association in 1896; President of the Philadelphia Neurological Society for two years; President of the Psychiatric Society for one year; Member of the American College of Physicians in 1923.

He was also elected a member of the following foreign societies: The Société de Neurologie de Paris, 1908; the Royal Medical Society of Budapest, 1909; the neurological section of the Royal Society of Medicine of London; the Psychiatric and Neurological Society of Vienna, 1911; the Society of

Physicians of Vienna, 1921. He was decorated Chevalier of the French Legion of Honor, 1923.

As final illustrations of Dr. Dercum's intellectual activity may be mentioned the following works relating to Neurology and allied topics which were prepared during his professional career. Edited a Text Book of Nervous Diseases by American authors, 1895, 1056 pp.; Rest, Suggestion, and Other Therapeutic Measures in Nervous and Mental Diseases, 1917, 395 pp.; Clinical Manual of Mental Diseases, 1913, 2d edition, 1917, 425 pp.; Hysteria and accident Compensation; Nature of Hystgeria and the lesson of the post-litigation results, 1916, 120 pp.; The Physiology of Mind, an interpretation based on biological, morphological, physical, and chemical considerations, 1922, 2nd edition, 1925, 287 pp.; Biology of the Internal Secretions, 1924, 241 pp..

In 1892 Dr. Dercum married Elizabeth De Haven Comly, a member of an old Philadelphia family. Mrs. Dercum and two daughters, Mrs. Samuel W. Mifflin and Miss Mary De Haven Dercum, survive.

As previously stated Dr. Dercum resigned his professorial duties in June 1925 with the view of devoting himself to the study of biological problems which had occupied his attention during leisure hours for may years. A few months previous to this time however Dr. Charles D. Walcott and Dr. Dercum had been elected President and Vice-President respectively of the American Philosophical Society both of whom had been members for many years.

In 1927 February 9, the distinguished President of the Society Dr. Walcott unexpectedly died much to the regret of the members generally as his death was regarded as a distinct loss to the interests of the Society.

At the Annual Meeting of the Society held April 1927 Dr. Dercum was chosen by the members to succeed Dr. Walcott as President. This great honor was profoundly appreciated and for four years, to the hour of his death he performed the duties incidental to the office with distinction and with great benefit to the Society.

Surveying his achievements during the four years of his presidency the most striking was his successful effort in raising the necessary funds for the erection of a new, more suitable and commodious building for the Society which the passing of the years, the growth of the library, the shifting of the population seemed to make most desirable.

For some years the members of the Society had entertained a dream of a new home for the Society in which could be housed in absolute safety the extensive collection of priceless relics of the builders of this nation, the valuable portraits and busts of its Presidents and many of its members, the rare historical letters and manuscripts, the thousands of old and many irreplaceable historical volumes of the library, all of which are among the cherished possessions of the Society.

For years it had been apparent that a Society for promoting useful knowledge owed it to scholarly research to provide increased facilities for readers and research students of the early history of our nation. But alas! the means for accomplishing this desirable end were wanting.

Very shortly after Doctor Dercum's election to the Presidency he inaugurated and directed in conjunction with his associates the movement which resulted in the securing of a fund sufficient to transmute the vague long-cherished dream into a rapidly-approaching reality. There can be no doubt that in doing so he initiated a new era in the life of the American Philosophical Society.

The current affairs of the Society received his constant attention and enlisted his active interest. By unceasing personal effort he brought to the meetings eminent scholars as speakers and auditors. As a result, the meetings increased in interest and significance. He himself contributed four papers to the Proceedings of the Society, viz.: "The Origin and Activities of the American Philosophical Society,"

"The Dynamic Factor in Evolution," "On the Nature of Thought and its Limitation" and "Non-Living and Living Matter."

Death came suddenly to him, seated in Benjamin Franklin's chair, as he presided over the first session of the General Meeting of the Society for 1931. Surrounded by many of his scientific colleagues and friends and the portraits of many of America's great men who had bequeathed this Society to successive generations, he had just spoken concerning the progress and the ambitions which the Society entertains and expressed the belief that these ambitions had every prospect of being realized. It seemed to be his bequest to the present generation. His memory will be gratefully and affectionately cherished.

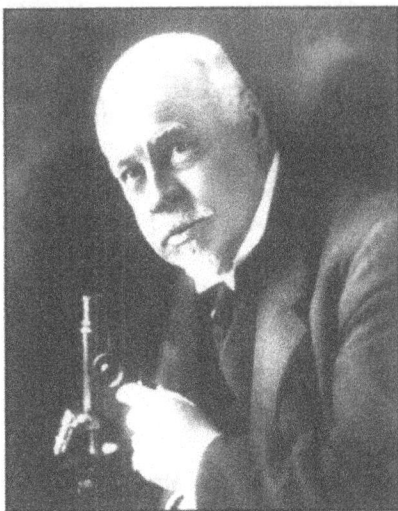

WILLIAM HENRY WELCH

1850–1934 (APS 1896)

Memoir by Simon Flexner

Doctor William H. Welch died in Baltimore on April 30, 1934, at the age of eighty-four years, and after a remarkable career in medicine extending over sixty years, of which fifty were spent at the Johns Hopkins University where, in succession, he was Professor of Pathology from 1884 to 1916, Director of the School of Hygiene and Public Health from 1917 to 1926, and Professor of the History of Medicine from 1926 to 1931. Upon his final retirement from active professional duties he became Professor Emeritus in the Institute of the History of Medicine which is associated with the splendid library that bears his name.

Doctor Welch was descended from a family of doctors—his grandfather, father, and his father's four brothers all having been physicians. His father stands out notably among the others, not only as a leading and successful practitioner, but as a socially minded member of the community of Norfolk, Connecticut, which held him in the highest esteem.

He served his state in its legislature, and his country in Congress, and after his death a memorial fountain was erected in his honor beside the house in which he lived and in which his even more gifted son was born. This house now carries a bronze tablet placed there on the occasion of the eightieth birthday of William H. Welch, as part of the international celebration of the event held in Washington, in which the President of the United States participated.

The last mentioned occasion was unique in the history of a scientist, for not only were the addresses of the President and of Doctor Welch carried by radio throughout the world, but in many other cities in the United States, in England, France, and Germany, as well as in Peiping and Tokyo, coincident celebrations were held.

Doctor Welch was graduated from Yale College in 1870, and from the College of Physicians and Surgeons (now Columbia University), New York, in 1874. Eighteen months were spent as intern at Bellevue Hospital, partly before graduation in medicine. The two years from 1876 to 1878 were passed in Germany, working under such masters as Waldeyer in anatomy, Hoppe-Seyler in physiological chemistry, Ludwig in physiology, and von Recklinghausen and Cohnheim in pathology.

The original purpose was to follow the clinics in internal medicine, with neurology as a special field of study. As laboratory training in the fundamental medical sciences was in this country all but absent from the medical curriculum of the period, Doctor Welch followed a natural bent in seeking this foundation in Germany. A strong impulse to this course came also from the experiences at Bellevue Hospital under Doctor Francis Delafield, whose devotion to human pathology was as unusual as his knowledge was profound.

As the two years gradually came to a close, Doctor Welch's interests became more certainly centered on pathology as a career, although the outlook was sufficiently discouraging. The six years following the return from Germany were spent partly in private practice, which provided the necessary economic support, and partly as professor of pathology at the University and Bellevue Hospital Medical College, where the first real courses in that subject ever offered in America were given.

Doctor Welch's European reputation, as well as his success as a teacher and investigator in New York, brought his definitive opportunity when in 1884 he was called to the Johns Hopkins University as Professor of Pathology and as advisor to the president and trustees in the selection of a staff for the Johns Hopkins Hospital (then under construction) and the faculty of the associated medical school supposedly soon to be established.

The immediate need felt by Doctor Welch was for the new bacteriology which, under the influence of the amazing discoveries appearing in rapid succession from the laboratory of Robert Koch, promised to transform the science and art of medicine. Hence the next year was spent in Berlin in work with Koch and his pupils, so that on his return to Baltimore in 1885, Doctor Welch was in position to offer a combined course in pathology, which embraced morbid anatomy, bacteriology, and pathological physiology, or experimental medicine.

No such comprehensive course of instruction and research had previously been undertaken even in Germany, and the remarkable success with which it was conducted by Doctor Welch was a tribute to his extraordinary learning and versatility, and his great gifts as a teacher. Doctor Welch's career as teacher, investigator, and educator may be divided into three periods, of which the longest is that devoted to the pursuit of pathology, extending actually from the Bellevue internship in 1875 to the retirement form the chair of pathology in Baltimore in 1916—approximately forty years.

The Baltimore professorship itself covered thirty years, and this in turn can be divided into two parts: that from 1885 to 1900, in which Doctor Welch devoted his energies chiefly to the laboratory; and another from 1900 to 1916, during which heavy and unremitting demands were made on his time by other institutions seeking his aid in the struggle upwards toward improved curricula and provision for research, which the successful example of the Johns Hopkins Medical School had made imperative.

Doctor Welch yielded graciously to these demands and accepted the sacrifice of his own dominant passion in the interests of the general and, as he believed greater educational good. Undoubtedly, a major effect of his wider influence was the creation of careers for scientifically trained men, which in the next quarter of a century was to bring American medical education and research abreast of the highest European models.

145

A measure of Doctor Welch's activity as an investigator in pathology may be found in a partial list of articles based on studies made in Europe and America during his more strictly laboratory years. They include such subjects as pulmonary edema, hemorrhagic infarction, thrombosis and embolism, glomerulo-nephritis, adaptation in pathological processes, hog cholera and swine plague, acute lobar pneumonia, diphtheria, wound infection, typhoid bacilli carriers, and Bacillus aerogenes capsulatus, nov. spec.

The next fifteen years were given over in considerable part to the wider public service already alluded to. Doctor Welch became the apostle, as it were, of the newer medicine in its application to teaching and research; and his trusteeship on such boards as that of the Carnegie Institution of Washington, the International Health Board, and similar institutions, enabled him to extend his wisely constructive influence into the field of general science and public health.

The extent and variety of these activities may be indicated by selected titles from his many public addresses, among which are: Advantages of the union of medical school and university; advancement of medical education; higher medical education and its need of endowment; the material needs of medical education; the benefits of the endowment of medical research; the position of natural science in education, medicine and the university; the medical curriculum; the relation of the hospital to medical education and research; the present position of medical education, its development and great needs for the future.

The second main period of Doctor Welch's career was devoted to the creation of the School of Hygiene and Public Health in Baltimore. For this there was no adequate model; he conceived the school as something commensurate with the important position which the public health held in the esteem of informed and forward-looking men. As he had long pondered the matter and it had been the subject of some of his impressive addresses, he set himself the task of outlining an institution in which instruction and research should be equally represented. Fortunately, this model was realized in practice; it became the standard toward which European countries strove when opportunity presented itself, as was presently the case, for the establishment of similar schools of their own.

A few titles will suffice to indicate the part which Doctor Welch played in arousing and guiding opinion in this country regarding the public health: Modes of infection; considerations concerning some external sources of infection in their bearing on preventive medicine; sanitation in relation to the poor; relation of laboratories to public health; duties of a hospital to public health; child welfare; the significance of the great frequency of tuberculous infection in early life in the prevention of disease, and what may be expected from more effective application of preventive measures against tuberculosis.

Another activity which brought large rewards was the part that Doctor Welch played in presiding at and attending congresses on hygiene at home and abroad, and in lending the weight of his name and great prestige to the public health movement.

We now come to the concluding period of Doctor Welch's rich and varied life. He retired from the directorship of the School of Hygiene and Public Health in 1926, at the age of seventy-six. But this gesture, like that of his retirement from the chair of pathology ten years earlier, was one of form only; it did not mean release from academic responsibilities, but rather the assumption of new duties. The new undertaking was one which appealed strongly to Doctor Welch's intellectual predilection and fell in with convictions which he had long held, namely that "the study of the history of medicine, notwithstanding its interest and value, is a study much neglected." The opportunity arose to put into effect this belief, and none other than Doctor Welch was available to assume the task.

As a memorial to Doctor Welch's extraordinary services as a pioneer and innovator in medical education and research, a magnificent medical library was about to be erected and endowed, and the Institute of the History of Medicine, which he had hoped might some day come into existence, was now to be incorporated into the library bearing his name—its proper and most favorable home.

A digression is justified at this point. Doctor Welch's compelling impulses toward scientific medicine revealed themselves early in his career. He had no more than graduated from Yale and entered the medical college than he left the latter, to return to New Haven for a year of advanced study in chemistry. This strong love for the fundamentals of knowledge was no passing fancy; it displayed itself again in Germany, when Doctor Welch sacrificed the clinic for the laboratory, through which he acquired the wide training and knowledge that were to enable him to lecture with a rare fascination and with equal facility on histology, pathology, bacteriology, and physiology, and to conduct and inspire research in all these branches.

The encyclopedic breadth of his mind carried him also into literature, history, and the arts; and those who were so fortunate as to become his companions and friends found his geniality of person, charm of manner, and conversational gifts irresistible. Thus the history of medicine, which in reality for him was the history of science and civilization, was an absorbing avocation from his early manhood. To have had the opportunity at the close of an eventful life of generous length to add to his achievements the founding of the Institute of the History of Medicine was one of those fitting rewards that come oftener in romance than in reality.

But was not Doctor Welch's life one long intellectual and spiritual romance? To find a counterpart, we are driven back to the Renaissance era, and the comparison of Doctor Welch's versatile gifts with those of Leonardo da Vinci is not merely a fanciful idea. Had Leonardo been born into the nineteenth century, he might well have been a scientist; and had Doctor Welch been born into the fifteenth, he would by the same tokens have chosen the arts and literature in which to nourish his omnivorous mind.

We may conclude this brief sketch of Doctor Welch's career with selected titles of addresses which illustrate his interest in scientific, historical subjects: The evolution of modern scientific laboratories; the influence of anesthesia upon medical science; some of the conditions which have influenced the development of American medicine, especially during the past century; the interdependence of medicine and other sciences of nature; Rudolph Virchow, pathologist; works and portraits to illustrate epochs in the history of medicine; the times of Vesalius; contributions of Vesalius other than anatomical; two physician-economists, Sir William Petty, 1623–1687, and Francois Quesney, 1694–1774; the development of English medicine as represented in a collection of medical portraits; the influence of English medicine upon American medicine in its formative period; William Wood Gerhard, and the differentiation of typhus and typhoid fevers; the fiftieth anniversary of the discovery of the tubercle bacillus; and the history of pathology.

EDITORS' NOTE

No one was better qualified than Simon Flexner to write this memoir. Yet it skips over what many would view as the most important aspect of a career which resulted in Welch being called the Dean of American Medicine. Not mentioned by Flexner is that he was also the first Dean of the Johns Hopkins School of Medicine. Even before the medical school opened he recruited to staff the new hospital a group of young clinicians who would soon be recognized as the best in American medicine: William Osler in Medicine, Howard Kelly in Gynecology and William Halsted in Surgery. He then appointed equally outstanding scientists and teachers for the Medical School including Franklin Mall, William T. Councilman, John Abel, William H. Howell, George Frederick Barker, William S. Thayer, Simon Flexner, Alexander Abbott and many others. Virtually all of them (except for the surgeons) became APS members. They and other Welch protégés became leaders of American medicine in other schools as well as Hopkins.

Welch's relationship with his chosen surgeon is a special story. Welch brought his friend Halsted from New York, rescuing him from a debilitating cocaine addicted state to make him Hopkins Chief of Surgery. Halsted went on to become American's greatest surgeon. Welch and Osler guarded for their lifetimes the secret that Halsted never overcame his need for narcotics.

Also missing from the memoir is reference to Welch's eccentricities and secret life. Welch was extremely personable. He socialized freely and was much beloved by his students and colleagues. Unlike his friend Halsted who was a recluse Welch loved excursions to garish seashore resorts such as Atlantic City. Little of his activities on these holidays was known. There were no women in his life. Harvey Cushing, in his Pulitzer Prize- winning biography of William Osler, suggested that Welch was homosexual, though offering no evidence. Lovingly referred to as Popsie, a limerick popular among the students tells the story:

Nobody knows where Popsie eats,
Nobody knows where Popsie sleeps,
Nobody knows whom Popsie keeps,
But Popsie.

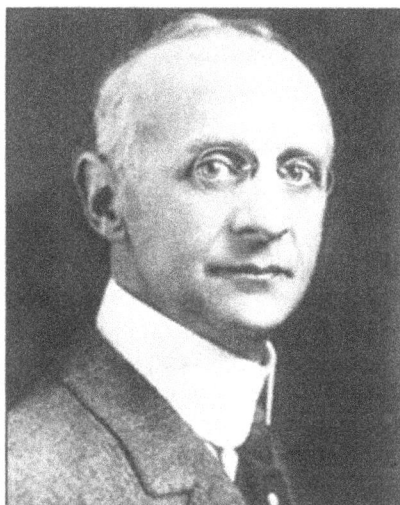

SIMON FLEXNER

1863–1946 (APS 1901)

Memoir by S. Bayne-Jones

Simon Flexner was born in Louisville, Kentucky, on March 25, 1863, and died in New York City on May 2, 1946. Within the eighty-three years spanned by his life, modern scientific medicine developed phenomenally abroad and in this country. He came into the field as a graduate in medicine at about the time when the new era of the discoveries of Pasteur, Koch, and a host of brilliant investigators in Europe had reached a peak, carrying bacteriology, immunology, and pathology to heights from which the topography of the biology of disease could be seen.

Within the half century of his own work in experimental medicine the extraordinary growth of medical science in the United States took place, constituting a revolution in thought and action in America, the "heroic age of American medicine," as Dr. Flexner described it in his biography of Dr. William H. Welch. An able investigator, constant in his faith that advance in biological knowledge would increase freedom from disease, a wise director and adviser, Dr. Flexner was one of the great figures of those times. Through the part he played in some of the largest undertakings of the period, he was one of the makers of the history of this new era.

Simon Flexner, the fourth son of Morris Flexner, a merchant, and Esther Abraham Flexner, was one of a large family of seven brothers and two sisters. The troubles of the Civil War followed by the depression of the early seventies made it necessary for the boys to earn money to help meet the family expenses. While still in public school Simon Flexner went to work as an errand boy in a drugstore. It is reported that in the drugstore he found a microscope which started his interest in the laboratory aspects of medicine.

To improve himself he graduated from a school of pharmacy. Later, while still serving as a clerk for a druggist, who was wise enough to let him take time off to attend lectures, he studied medicine at the Medical Department of the University of Louisville, and graduated there with the degree of M.D. in 1889, at the age of twenty-six.

Of his medical training Dr. Flexner wrote: "A druggist in Louisville, I had studied medicine at an old fashioned school, the University of Louisville. I had not attempted to practice, but had used Delafield and Prudden's book, as well as some other simple texts, to teach myself a little pathology. My preparation was thus most rudimentary." However rudimentary his formal preparation may have been, he had a feeling for pathology and a straightforward interest in that field. His first papers, published in the Louisville medical journal The American Practitioner and News in the first year after his graduation, were on clinical chemistry, laboratory diagnosis, and anatomical pathology. They show that by 1890 he was familiar with the Bulletin of the Johns Hopkins Hospital and was well aware of discoveries made abroad, as he writes about the tubercle bacillus, the bacillus of typhoid, the gonococcus, and Laveran's protozoan (the malarial parasite), and other pathogenic microorganisms.

At this time The American Practitioner and News like the New Orleans Medical and Surgical Journal was full of abstracts of foreign articles and in almost every issue published a "London letter" or a "Paris letter." Indeed, these Southern medical journals carried so much medical and scientific news that any discerning and intelligent reader of the time would become well informed and would find plenty of ideas and connections for his work. It is no belittlement of the great and effective advances that stemmed from Baltimore and the Northeastern seaboard region to point out the simultaneous inflow of new knowledge into the South from foreign sources.

No doubt this medical intelligence influenced and served Dr. Flexner well. He appears to have entered into correspondence with Dr. Welch first through seeking opinions on "anomalous tumors." Dr. Flexner's selection of pathology as his main interest and his letters to Dr. Welch in 1889 and 1890 were momentous for the lives of both men and for medical science. In the fall of 1890 he went to Baltimore eager to work in Welch's laboratory. At this time he had no great plans for the future, intending on his return home to eke out a living from pathology and bacteriology. Within a few months Dr. Welch had recognized Dr. Flexner's gift for investigation, and through an influence more subtle than is indicated by such words as "inspiration and guidance," set him on the course of his career. Thus began a life-long friendship which was of the greatest consequence to their separate and joint attainments, as it was also to the advancement of science.

The next nine years were a happy and productive period for Dr. Flexner in teaching and research at the Pathological Laboratory at Johns Hopkins. In a somewhat paradoxical manner he throve systematically in the laissez-faire life of the place, investigating typhoid fever, pancreatitis, tuberculosis, and other infections, learning as he went and contributing to basic knowledge by his own experiments. In 1895 he was made Assistant Professor of Pathology and in 1899 he was promoted to Professor of Pathologic Anatomy at the Johns Hopkins University Medical School.

When the United States Army Board for the investigation of tropical diseases in the Philippine Islands was formed in 1899, under the presidency of Dr. Richard Pearson Strong, Dr. Flexner was selected to assist with the pathological and bacteriological work. Entering upon this expedition with enthusiasm he utilized every opportunity for investigation of diseases in different strange places. He studied plague in Hong Kong and in the Philippines discovered the important type of dysentery bacillus which became famous as the Flexner bacillus.

In 1899 Dr. Flexner was appointed Professor of Pathology at the University of Pennsylvania and he took up that position on his return from the Philippines in 1900. At the same time he was appointed Director of the Ayer Clinical Laboratory and Pathologist of the University Hospital. He entered upon teaching and research with enthusiasm and soon had around him a group of promising student associates among whom was Dr. Hideyo Noguchi. Many problems of infectious diseases were attacked and an important line of investigation was opened by his work on toxalbumins, the biochemical constitution of snake venoms and the preparation and study of anti-venoms.

In 1901 he was elected to membership in the American Philosophical Society. During the two years from 1900 to 1902 he demonstrated his capacity to organize and conduct an important laboratory and strengthened his position as an original investigator, now internationally recognized. During the same time events were impending which contained his destiny as a leader in great new developments in experimental medicine in America.

The beginning of these events was probably the conversations which the Reverend Frederick T. Gates, about 1897, had with Mr. John D. Rockefeller about his conviction that medicine could hardly hope to become a science until it should be endowed and until qualified men could devote themselves to uninterrupted study and investigation, entirely independent of practice, and that the best way to do this was to establish an institute for medical research in the United States. The Rockefeller Institute for Medical Research, founded in 1901 by Mr. John D. Rockefeller and supported thereafter by large gifts from himself and Mr. John D. Rockefeller, Jr., was the final embodiment of these discussions.

The beginnings were cautious and slow. The first funds were expended in grants-in-aid. Soon it was realized that a central laboratory would be needed and that a director would be required. The first selection for this post was Dr. Theobald Smith, who as Dr. Flexner has written "had from the first been regarded as the natural choice for the director of the laboratory…since he had been proved America's leading investigator by his brilliant investigations of Texas fever of cattle, which demonstrated conclusively the principle of insect transmission of disease, thus opening a new chapter in the study of parasitology."

Dr. Smith declined the directorship because he felt it would be better to have as director a man thoroughly identified with advances in human pathology. Dr. Simon Flexner then became the unanimous choice of the board of advisers, composed of Drs. Welch, Smith, Herter, and Prudden, and he was invited to accept this appointment in the spring of 1902. Dr. Flexner accepted in June 1902 after thorough study of the situation and examination of his own prospects.

In accepting the directorship of the Institute's laboratory, Dr. Flexner had to consider giving up an assured academic position for one of indefinite tenure, and exchanging an established department for an adventure into experimental medicine in a new laboratory which would depend for its future entirely upon its output. He was happy at the University of Pennsylvania. He had many misgivings about the proposed change. Modestly he was doubtful about his competence to conduct a purely research laboratory. What would happen if the prop of teaching was wholly removed? What about tenure and what would happen at the end of the ten years for which support of the new laboratory had been pledged?

He was shy about the great commercial city of New York which was said to be cold to scientific medicine. The prospect seemed to be full of terrors. In accepting the directorship of the Rockefeller Institute of Medical Research in 1902, Dr. Flexner showed characteristically great courage. He had vision and audacity. While realizing that the future of the Institute would depend upon initial success, he laid broad plans for fundamental research. Convinced that the future of scientific medicine lay in basic research and trusting in the means to conduct studies and to assemble the best men to make them, he committed his life to this adventure. For the rest of his years the Rockefeller Institute became largely his life.

This is not the place to review the scientific contributions of the distinguished members of the Institute or its organization and physical growth. It is to be said, however, that the staff, their ways of work, both independent and directed, the organization and the great buildings were all reflections of Dr. Flexner's ideals, philosophy, methods, and innate directive power. Departing from the structure of the existing prototypes, the Pasteur and Koch Institutes, he evolved an organization best suited to his ideas. This organization resembled that of a university, with the prime emphasis on research, but providing also for education and training.

His vision of the unity of pathology gradually took final form. The first small laboratory in a rented building at 127 East 50th Street in New York, opened in 1904, became in 1906 the great Central Laboratory located in the tract of land overlooking the East River at 66th Street. The Hospital of the Rockefeller Institute for Medical Research, adjacent to the Central Laboratory, was opened in 1910. In 1914 the Department of Animal Pathology was created at Princeton, New Jersey, and in 1931 the Laboratory of Plant Pathology was added at Princeton.

Thus was provision made in one organization for the study of disease as it occurs in all the main orders of living things. In 1933, perhaps thinking of this organization, Dr. Flexner said: "There are no closed compartments in nature into which man, animals and plants can be separately placed. All are related organically and, as we may say, united physiologically and pathologically. No essential biological division exists between men and the lower animals and plants, whether in respect to health or to disease."

In 1904, when the Rockefeller Institute for Medical Research was barely under way a severe epidemic of cerebrospinal meningitis struck New York City and the adjacent country. Dr. Flexner immediately devoted himself and the resources of the Institute to an attack on the problems of meningococcal infection. A long series of valuable studies followed, the most notable being his production of a serum for use in the treatment of the disease. The use of this serum reduced the case fatality rate by half and until the advent of the sulfanilamide drugs was the most hopeful treatment.

The epidemic of poliomyelitis which struck the eastern states in 1908 aroused Dr. Flexner's keenest interest. At a time when relatively little was known about viruses he made this infection a major field for study. In 1909, through independent research, and at about the same time as Landsteiner's discovery abroad, he and Lewis succeeded in transmitting the disease to monkeys and showed that the infection could be produced not only by intraperitoneal inoculation, but also by subcutaneous, intravenous, and intraneural inoculation, and he proved that the virus occurred in the nasopnaryngeal mucus and that monkeys could be infected by the intranasal application of virus containing material.

This pointed to the respiratory transmission of the disease and, until others showed that the virus occurs in feces and sewage, it stood as the only approximately proved mode of transmission. The facts he discovered have been basic contributions. The problems of poliomyelitis held his interest for the rest of his life.

The final major problem that Dr. Flexner took up was the intricate one of experimental epidemiology, which he approached through the methods of observation of "mouse-villages," the effects of herd immunity and the rise and fall of outbreaks of infection following the introduction of susceptibles or newly infected individuals into the animal populations.

From the first, education and dissemination of knowledge was one of the aims of the Rockefeller Institute for Medical Research. It was natural, therefore, that Dr. Flexner took satisfaction in the transfer of the Journal of Experimental Medicine from Johns Hopkins, where it had been started by Dr. Welch and others, after discussions lasting over two years from 1893 to 1895, to the Rockefeller Institute for Medical Research in October 1904. Dr. Flexner undertook the editorship and served as editor until he died in 1946. The qualities of his editorship, as summarized in the July 1946 issue of the journal, are so much the character of the man that the passage is quoted.

Dr. Flexner respected the individuality of authors.... He was no believer in the editorial reconditioning of papers nor did he become intolerant of certain words met too often, as is the unhappy way of editors. His own style was pellucid, and simplicity and clarity meant so much to him that stylistic adventurings made him uneasy, though he countenanced them for the greater good. Indeed he was liberal to everything except repetitive work and trivial discovery.

Devoted with unvarying singleness of purpose to the Rockefeller Institute for Medical Research, Dr. Flexner restricted his activities in outside affairs as much as possible. There were however, notable exceptions. He visited Europe on numerous occasions. A notable trip abroad was in 1911 when he, the first American so honored, received the Cameron Prize and delivered distinguished lectures.

In the First World War he was commissioned in the Medical Corps and went abroad to improve the laboratory service of the Army. Through years he served on the Advisory Board of the American Red Cross. Year after year at legislative hearings he successfully defended medical progress against the anti-vivisectionists. For years he was a member of the Public Health Council of New York State and became its chairman.

Two of his greatest contributions made outside of the Institute were connected with the Rockefeller Foundation. In 1913 he became one of the charter members of the Rockefeller Foundation and through the years that followed he exerted an extraordinary influence in the group of strong and positive men who constituted its board. The establishment of the National Research Council fellowships in physics and chemistry and in the biological sciences was based upon plans which he initiated and developed.

In 1915 he was one of the members of the China Medical Board Commission which was sent to China to survey medical conditions and to develop plans for the promotion of Western medicine in China. The establishment of the Peking Union Medical College was largely a result of his creative mind.

In 1935, at the age of seventy-two, Dr. Flexner retired as Director of the Rockefeller Institute for Medical Research. Dr. Herbert S. Gasser, his successor, has described the becoming manner in which Dr. Flexner after his retirement cut himself off completely from the administrative affairs of the Institute. Still energetic and keenly interested he continued during the remaining years of his life to write scientific papers, and devoted himself particularly to the writing, in collaboration with his son, Dr. James Thomas Flexner, of the biography of his great friend Dr. Welch. This work appeared in 1941 under the title: William Henry Welch and the Heroic Age of American Medicine. It was a fitting final volume for his life history as for the great leader and his age.

Shortly after his retirement Dr. Flexner became Eastman Professor at Oxford University. This was only one of many honors that he received during his life-time. Eighteen universities in this country and abroad gave him honorary degrees. He was a Fellow of Balliol College, Oxford. He was a member of the National Academy of Sciences, Foreign Member of the Royal Society of London, Foreign

Associate of the Institute of France, and Commander of the French Legion of Honor. He was a member of numerous scientific bodies in the United States, South America, and Europe.

In 1903 Dr. Flexner married Miss Helen Whitall Thomas of Bryn Mawr, Pennsylvania. They had two sons, William Welch Flexner and James Thomas Flexner. Dr. Flexner was a medium sized man, rather frail looking, with fine features and fine hands. He was modest, apparently almost shy. His soft-toned voice was rarely, if ever, raised in pitch. He was gentle but firm, courageous and steadfast. Within his personality there was a force which seemed not to need a large physique. These are impressions. The tributes of his intimates were paid in eloquent descriptions by Dr. Peyton Rous, Dr. Herbert S. Gasser, Mr. Raymond Fosdick, Judge Learned Hand, and Mr. John D. Rockefeller, Jr. at the memorial exercises held in the library of the Rockefeller Institute for Medical Research on June 12, 1946. After telling of his accomplishments they spoke of his courage and attractive leadership, his simplicity and modesty, his gentleness and force, and his kindliness and wisdom.

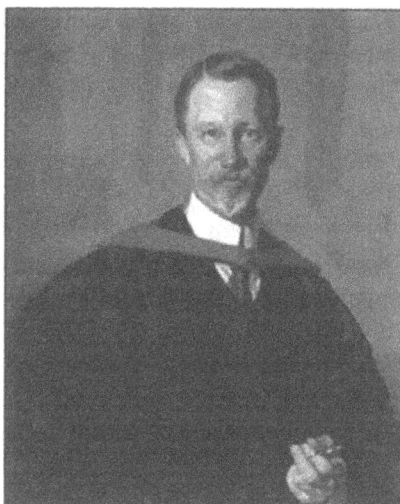

WILLIAM HENRY HOWELL

1860–1945 (APS 1903)

Memoir by Joseph Erlanger

William Henry Howell, son of George Henry and Virginia Magruder Howell, was born in Baltimore, February 20, 1860. His education was acquired entirely in his native city. During his senior year at high school (the "Baltimore City College") he became assistant to the professor of physics and chemistry and did not complete the course. Nevertheless, he was admitted to the Johns Hopkins University where he took the chemical-biological course with the intention of preparing himself for a career in medicine.

Upon his graduation in 1881 he was awarded a graduate scholarship and two years later a fellowship, and consequently forwent his original intention and became a candidate for the Ph.D. degree. However, while pursuing his graduate studies he carried extramural courses in human anatomy at the medical school of the University of Maryland and attended medical clinics there. He was granted the Ph.D. degree in 1884, the title of his dissertation being "The Origin of Fibrin Formed in the Coagulation of the Blood."

The following year he was appointed Chief Assistant in the department of his teacher, Newell Martin, and during the five succeeding years was rapidly advanced to the rank of Associate Professor of Biology. In the latter capacity he gave the lectures in animal physiology. In 1889 he accepted appointment as Lecturer in Physiology in the University of Michigan and after one year, at age thirty, became Professor of Physiology there. In 1892 he was called to Harvard University as Associate Professor of Physiology in the department of Henry Pickering Bowditch and in 1893 he returned to his alma mater as the first Professor of Physiology in the Medical School, a post he held until 1918. During this period he served for twelve years, from 1899 until 1911, as Dean of the Medical School in succession to Dr. Welch, the first dean.

155

When the School of Hygiene and Public Health of the Johns Hopkins University was founded in 1918 he severed his connection with the Medical School to accept appointment as Assistant Director and Professor of Physiology in the School of Hygiene. Eight years later he succeeded Dr. Welch as Director of that school.

He was retired in 1931, but was provided with a laboratory by the university and, with funds supplied, first, by a research foundation, and subsequently, from the fluid research fund of the Medical School he continued to experiment almost to the day of his death, though he knew he had arterial sclerosis and was having some heart attacks. At 5:00 A.M. on February 6, 1945, he was seized with a severe attack and died almost immediately, a few days before his eighty-fifth birthday. His mind retained its pristine clearness to the end.

Throughout his career Dr. Howell's prime interest was research. The earliest of his approximately eighty scientific papers dealt with the heart beat and with certain aspects of the physiology of blood; indeed, coagulation of the blood and the physiological action of the salts of the blood can be regarded as his major fields of research. One of his first contributions consisted in showing that serum albumin is not essential to the nourishment of the heart, as had been asserted by European physiologists, but that it was the inorganic content of their perfusion solutions that had maintained the beat of the heart.

His interest in salt action suggested to him the possibility that cardiac inhibition might be due to the liberation of diffusible potassium in the heart, and his experiments demonstrated that it is. Later, Loewi found that acetylcholine also is liberated by vagus stimulation; and since atropine stops the action of acetylcholine but not that of potassium Loewi concluded that acetylcholine is the inhibitor. More recently, Lenhartz showed that acetylcholine liberates potassium, but not in the presence of atropine. It would seem, therefore, that potassium is the actual inhibitor of the heart and that Howell should be credited with the first demonstration of chemical transmission of nerve action.

Howell made important contributions in the field of circulation and endocrine physiology also, but his name is most conspicuously identified with the process of blood coagulation. Among his more significant findings in this field may be mentioned the isolation of some of the more important chemical factors that play a role in coagulation, such, for example, as cephalin and heparin. At the age of seventy-seven he published a finding of great interest, namely, that in extrauterine life blood platelets, a source of cephalin, are formed primarily in the lungs. Just prior to his death he was busily investigating a new blood coagulant. In 1905 he published his Text-book of Physiology for Medical Students and Physicians; it was in its fourteenth edition at the time of his death.

The position Dr. Howell occupied in American physiology may be best evaluated by the recognition accorded him by his colleagues. He was one of the twenty-eight charter members of the American Physiological Society and read the first paper at the first meeting of that society. He was its fourth president and was younger by many years than were his predecessors at the time of their incumbency. He was reelected to the office five times. He was chosen by American physiologists to be the president of the first and only International Physiological Congress to meet in the Americas. He was editor of the American Textbook of Physiology (1896), the first cooperative effort of the kind by new world physiologists.

He was elected a member of the American Philosophical Society in 1903 and of the National Academy of Sciences in 1905. He held honorary memberships in the (British) Physiological Society, in the Società Italiana di Biologia Sperimentale and was a member of the Kaiserl Leopold-Carolin Deutsche Akademie der Naturforscher zu Halle. He was granted an honorary M.D. degree by the

University of Michigan in 1890, the Sc.D. degree by Yale University in 1911, and LL.D. degrees by Trinity College in 1901, by the University of Michigan in 1912, by Washington University in 1915 and by the University of Edinburgh in 1923.

Dr. Howell was one of the best loved of American physiologists. A kindly disposition and simplicity of manner endeared him to all who knew him well. He held firm but carefully weighed convictions which, however, were never obtruded on casual acquaintances. His strength of intellect, his wisdom, his moral fiber gave him the peace of mind and the sympathetic understanding of his fellow men that were so apparent to all who knew him.

He enjoyed particularly the simple things in life—the out-of-doors, sailing in particular, and the comradeship of his family. He possessed the ability to express his thoughts in conversation, in the classroom and before assemblages, whether scientific or general, with a directness and a simplicity of verbiage that invariably charmed his hearers. He will be remembered not only for his important contributions to physiology, as an inspiring teacher and as an able and considerate administrator, but equally for his fine personal attributes—a calm, simple philosophy of life and the ability to live in the light of that philosophy.

In 1887 Dr. Howell married Anne Janet Tucker of Baltimore. He is survived by three children: Janet Howell Clark, Ph.D., Dean of the Woman's College, University of Rochester, Roger Howell, Ph.D., Dean and Professor of Constitutional Law, University of Maryland, and Charlotte Teresa Hulburt, wife of Dr. E. O. Hulburt, Naval Research Laboratory, Washington, D. C., and by seven grandchildren and two great-grandchildren.

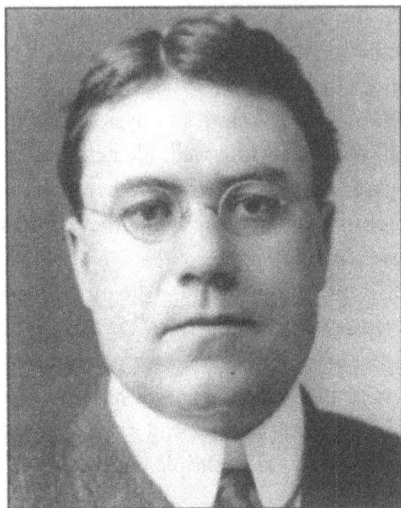

WALTER BRADFORD CANNON

1871–1945 (APS 1908)

Memoir by Alexander Forbes

If ever a man was self-made in the best sense of that phrase, it was Walter Bradford Cannon. In his admirable book, The Way of an Investigator, he has given an illuminating picture of his career from childhood to old age and especially of the lessons he learned from life. The story is told, not in the spirit of proud recital of achievement, but in simple, straightforward recognition of the help that he might give to others by passing these lessons on to them.

With a hereditary background of rugged pioneering stock, he was born at Prairie du Chien, Wisconsin, October 19, 1871. In this small town of the Middle West there was little tradition of scholarship in his early environment. He was encouraged to learn self-reliance in the use of hands and brain, to be diligent in the work of school or shop; but acceptance of religious dogma was expected of him rather than intellectual originality. The pioneer in him asserted itself in the noblest manner—a bent for philosophical thought which led him to study and ponder the works of Huxley, John Fiske, and others, to the dismay of family and clergy. Nothing could stop the growth of his mind or his zeal for learning and the quest for truth.

Yearning for higher education, he talked with a graduate of Harvard who awakened his eagerness to study at that university and, with the encouragement and help of a former teacher, he obtained a scholarship that enabled him to enter Harvard College in 1892. During the next eight years, aided only by scholarships, he worked his way through college and the Harvard Medical School.

Those who recall how largely the sons of prominent families in the big eastern cities dominated the human contacts in the undergraduate life of Harvard in the nineties can picture the lot of a boy from the Middle West, coming to work his way through college. So warm-hearted and human a boy as Walter Cannon may well have felt lonely and left out of it all.

Whether or not he felt that he was missing something of value, he was so engrossed in his studies and the arduous task of earning his living as well, that it did not disturb the growth of his mind and character. Few, if any, of his classmates can have suspected that in the quiet, unassuming student, unnoticed in their midst, was a truly great man in the making, a man destined to become one of the foremost leaders in the intellectual life of America.

Having to make his own way and struggle to support himself while acquiring his education, was in a way a handicap, but in another and perhaps larger way it was an advantage; the intrusion of bread-winning and financial worry into a career of scholarship was more than offset by his early training in the hard school of necessity. At least so we may judge from his graduation summa cum laude, his performance of epoch-making research in addition to routine duties as a medical student, and his rapid rise to eminence as a scholar, teacher, and citizen.

With the joyous zest of an eager explorer, he threw himself into his lifelong career of research in physiology, beginning as Instructor in the Harvard Medical School. His first field of inquiry was the mechanical factors of digestion, which is, in fact, the title of his first important book in 1911, embodying the results of fourteen years of research. Important as were the findings, it is probable that the ingenious new technique he devised for this research was the chief cause of his sudden rise to eminence and wide recognition in medical science.

His new method consisted of introducing the salts of a heavy metal into the food, thus rendering it opaque to x-rays, and then observing by fluoroscopy the nicely coordinated action of the muscles regulating the workings of the digestive tract. At one stroke he gave to physiology the first clear knowledge of the motor function of the digestive tract and to clinical medicine a new method of diagnosing disease in humans. It was during this part of his career, in 1906, that he succeeded Dr. Henry P. Bowditch as George Higginson Professor of Physiology in the Harvard Medical School.

With his genius for observing all manner of details and discerning their significance, Cannon noted the disturbing effects of emotional excitement on the digestive functions that were the object of his research. Instead of dismissing the troublesome disturbance as a mere nuisance, interfering with his program, he saw in it the starting point of a new and greater program of research—a broad survey of the effects of emotions on functional states in the animal body. These studies culminated in the publication in 1915 of Bodily Changes in Pain, Hunger, Fear and Rage, a book in which was developed the concept of emergency function of the sympathetic nervous system and especially of its potent end-organ, the adrenal medulla.

The publication of his original and far-reaching theory based on these observations gave rise to a controversy that is well described in chapter IX of The Way of an Investigator. In that chapter he draws some valuable lessons and shows how adverse criticism led him to devise new experiments and discover new truths until his main thesis was established beyond further controversy.

The First World War drew him into the struggle as a Medical Officer in the Army. In England and France he strove with the best experts that could be mobilized to solve the terrible problems of surgical shock in the wounded. Working now in the laboratory and now in the hospitals at the front, sometimes under heavy shellfire, he gave the best he had of mind, courage, and zeal to the saving of this life.

In this service he rose from First Lieutenant to Lieutenant Colonel at the close of the war, and in 1919 the British Government conferred on him the Cross of the Companion of the Bath for "Meritorious services for the Allied cause." In 1922 he received from our own Government the Distinguished Services Medal.

The results of his achievements were so great that in World War II he was made Chairman of a Committee on Shock and Transfusions of the National Research Council. In this capacity he resumed his beneficent work for the wounded, starting where he left off in 1921 and continuing throughout the war.

In 1919, resuming his duties as head of the Physiology Department at the Harvard Medical School, he solved the baffling problems of the emergency function of the adrenal medulla, and thus ended the long controversy. Once again, observations in one line of research suggested to him larger and more far-reaching generalizations; by scrutiny of a great variety of bodily functions he arrived at the concept of homeostasis which he defined as the maintenance of a steady state of the unstable substances within the body by means of nicely adjusted regulating systems that resist changes due to external disturbance.

Proper function requires that warm-blooded animals must maintain a nearly constant temperature within their bodies, and this need is met by a variety of heat-regulating mechanisms. And so it is with the concentration of salts and sugar and the acid-base equilibrium in the body fluids. In all these diverse functions he saw a common principle of self-regulation, and one of profound import to all life.

The last important chapter in his research career grew out of his scrutiny of a source of confusion in the course of his controversy on the adrenal function. A baffling phenomenon was subjected to careful and crucial experiments until it was proved that impulses in the sympathetic nerves cause the production of a substance that passes from the innervated structures into the blood stream and plays a part in the significant results of sympathetic excitation. From this grew a most important series of contributions on chemical mediation of the effects of nerve impulses, in which there was close and effective collaboration with his able colleague Arturo Rosenblueth, a master of electrical technique and of clear thinking.

On October 15, 1931, a notable gathering at Harvard paid tribute to Dr. Cannon on the occasion of his completion of twenty-five years as George Higginson Professor of Physiology. Distinguished speakers paid eloquent homage and praised his productive scholarship and especially his generous leadership in sending forth so many well-trained pupils to become leaders in physiology elsewhere. His response at the close of the exercises was gracious, modest, dignified and at the same time warmly appreciative of the esteem of his colleagues. The addresses delivered at the exercises held in Dr. Cannon's honor on October 15, 1931, and his response, together with his bibliography to date and lists of the positions he had held and honors bestowed ho him, were collected in a small volume entitled, "Walter Bradford Cannon 1906–1931", printed by the Harvard University Press.

In 1908 Dr. Cannon was elected a member of the American Philosophical Society in view of his distinction in the field of physiology, this being only one of the many recognitions which he received.

His life was a happy one. The freedom to seek truth and to serve greatly, earned by his own efforts, was what he most desired and what he had in full measure. The illness he suffered in later life was hard for him to bear, but still he enjoyed life and all the friendships that meant so much to him, and his genial cordiality remained to the end.

As a devoted champion of freedom, he took time from his studies to work hard and long for various causes that moved him to make the sacrifice. But, in spite of these digressions, his zeal and intellect combined to render his contribution to physiology the greatest, in my opinion, that has been achieved by any one man in America. The qualities of mind that made this possible were those of fertility, breadth of vision, and imagination, rather than powers of incisive reasoning. His mind was more like Darwin's or Huxley's than like those of Newton, LaPlace, or Maxwell.

He showed his own clear recognition of this in his chapter on "Fellowship in Exploration," in which he contrasts his own trend toward "synthetic or integrative physiology" with that of "analytic" physiologists. Even more important than the fertile quality of his mind was the dynamic effect of his boundless zeal and enthusiasm for the pursuit of knowledge.

His philosophy concerning the importance of science to human progress is summed up in the following sentence in his book "The Way of an Investigator" (p. 173). It is a timely reply to those who curse all science today because of the atomic bomb. "To resent the effects of science, to see it 'destroying all the simplicity and gentleness of life, all the beauty of the world—restoring barbarism under the mask of civilization, darkening men's minds and hardening their hearts,' is to admit an ability to face realities and make adjustments—precisely the functions which distinguish man, with his superior brain, from lower animals."

On October 1, 1945, Dr. Cannon died in his sleep. It is fortunate that he lived long enough to receive expressions of grateful appreciation of his book, "The Way of an Investigator", from many of his warm friends and admirers. To us who worked through the years in the laboratory with him in the most harmonious companionship, the sense of personal bereavement is overwhelming. The laboratory can never be the same, but we hope his spirit will long continue to live there.

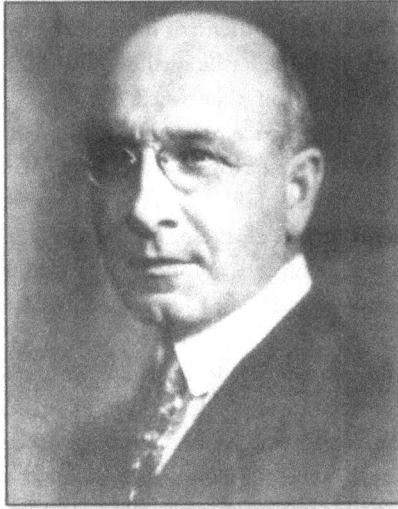

ALEXIS CARREL

1873–1944 (APS 1909)
Memoir by Simon Flexner

Dr. Alexis Carrel died in Paris on November 5, 1944, at the age of 71. He was educated in Lyon, France, his native city, taking his doctor of medicine degree in 1900. He had served as interne in the Lyon Hospital from 1896 to 1900, and as prosector from 1900 to 1904. Carrel seems from the outset to have been attracted to the laboratory rather than to the practice of surgery. In 1902, he published his first paper on the technique of the surgery of the blood vessels and the transplantation of organs, a subject which he was to make peculiarly his own, much to the enrichment of human surgery.

In 1904, he journeyed to Montreal to read a paper on this subject before the Second Congress of Medicine in the French Language of North America. In coming to America, Carrel must have had in mind the finding of more favorable opportunities for the pursuit of his experimental work. He did not, therefore, return to France, but attached himself to the physiological laboratory of the University of Chicago, where he spent two profitable years.

My attention was attracted to Carrel by a brief paper published in Science on October 13, 1905, in which he described the transplantation of a kidney in the dog, the renal artery being sutured to the carotid, the renal vein to the jugular, and the ureter to the oesophagus, the kidney continued to function. Carrel was little known in America at that time. At my invitation, he came to New York for an interview which led to a fellowship in the recently opened laboratory of The Rockefeller Institute, on which he entered in October 1906, just as the Institute moved from temporary quarters into its first laboratory building on the East River site. This circumstance made possible the assignment of space to him which he could develop according to his own ideas, a manifest advantage since his surgical work demanded the most rigid septic conditions.

162

Carrel was to spend the rest of his active scientific life in New York, returning to France during the annual summer vacation period. He was elected a member of The American Philosophical Society in 1909. The foundation of Carrel's work in experimental surgery rests on the perfection of the technique of vascular surgery, an almost unexplored field at the time; and he had the good fortune to see the methods which he devised applied to the saving of human life. Failure in vascular surgery arose mainly from the formation of a clot of blood (thrombus) in vessels operated upon, the chief causes of which were the injury inflicted upon the inner (endothelial) lining coat of the vessels, the entry of tissue juices into the vessels during operation causing the blood to clot, and from infection by bacteria. Carrel addressed himself to the correction of these errors. There can be no doubt that he possessed the essential intellectual perceptions, as well as the delicate skilled hands, of the master surgeon, which fitted him for the exacting work he had undertaken.

Carrel's surgical methods were novel and original. To control hemorrhage he dispensed with forceps, which crush the vessels, and replaced them by narrow linen bands; and for suturing the cut vessels, which involves injury to the endothelial inner lining, he employed very sharp, small, round needles, both needles and threads being coated with vaseline. When the vessels stretched by the needle thrusts contracted, the vaseline was rubbed off in the puncture holes and the wounded endothelium was covered, so that immediate contact with the circulating blood was prevented.

With this simple technique, it became possible to carry out successfully many diverse and often elaborate operations involving injury of blood vessels while still preserving the circulation. Injured vessels could be patched, excised parts could be replaced by vessels taken from other parts of the same animal, or from another animal of the same species, or even from a different species. And as preservation of the circulation was now accomplished, organs could be transplanted almost at will.

However, a limitation of the substitution method soon declared itself. The tissues and organs performing the higher functions of the body are specific for the species and also in lesser degree for the individual. A physiological result was obtainable in the replantation of organs in the same individual, sometimes with the transplantation of organs of another individual of the same species, and never with the transplantation of organs of a foreign species.

This is not the place to enter into the details of Carrel's many experiments and the degree to which they became applicable to human surgery. In 1912, the Nobel prize in medicine was awarded Carrel for his work on the suture of blood vessels and the transplantation of organs. In the address which he delivered on the occasion, he reviewed the work for which that great honor was conferred upon him. Carrel's experimental work directed his attention in an emphatic way to the restoration and reconstruction—reintegration—of injured tissues, a subject which is much in the mind of all surgeons. Carrel was prepared by training to follow these processes, both in their clinical aspects and in their manifestations as revealed by the microscope.

In this connection, he became deeply impressed with Ross G. Harrison's work on the development outside the body of the nervous tissues of the embryo frog. In the winter of 1908, Harrison gave a Harvey Lecture in New York, in which he described his culture method. Sometime later, Carrel spoke with me of going to Harrison's laboratory at Yale in order to learn the technique he employed. At my suggestion, his assistant, M. T. Burrows, was sent instead, a plan which proved especially profitable as Burrows remained long enough to carry out, under Harrison's guidance, the successful cultivation of tissues from the chicken embryo.

Carrel and Burrows set to work to cultivate the tissues of adult animals in vitro. The Harrison method was of beautiful simplicity: a fragment of tissue is placed in a drop of lymph or plasma on a cover-glass, inverted on a hollow glass slide, and observed under the microscope. They succeeded quickly in obtaining tissue cultures of connective tissue, cartilage, periosteum, bone and bone marrow, skin, cornea, buccal mucous membrane, thyroid and suprarenal glands, kidney, pancreas, testicle, and ovary, and in reactivating the cell growth by transferring the fragments into a fresh medium.

This was in 1910, and Carrel was to carry on the study of tissue cultures in his laboratory for the next quarter of a century, while the work was taken up and pursued actively elsewhere in this country and in Europe. In order to obtain cultures in indefinite series and in mass, the culture medium was modified by the addition of the juice of the embryo chick and in other ways. A strain of connective tissue derived from the heart of a chick embryo has been kept in active growth for more than thirty years, and pure strains of body cells have been obtained in much the same way as pure strain cultures of bacteria.

Carrel did not himself assemble the results of his work with tissue cultures, but his Danish pupil, Albert Fischer, published a book on the subject in Copenhagen in 1925, and his associate, Raymond C. Parker, a book in 1938. To the latter book, Carrel wrote a foreword in which his views on the importance of tissue cultures for the general physiologist are set forth. Tissue culture has been applied to the investigation of viruses, which require living cells for their propagation. Among the viruses cultivated are those of vaccinia, yellow fever, and rabies.

It is apparent that from his medical student days Carrel's mind was centered on the physiology of the tissues and organs from the surgical point of view. He entertained for a time the ambitious idea of substituting healthy organs for diseased ones in the human body, which the strict individual specificity of the organs themselves rendered impossible of accomplishment. But Carrel's absorption in the physiology of the separate organs was not abated by this failure. He had proceeded from the investigation of the complete organs to their parts in tissue culture, and in his final work he was to succeed with the devising of methods for the culture of whole organs, and thus to realize, at least in part, his early ambition.

Carrel's attempts to keep alive functioning organs removed from the body began with his work on visceral organisms in 1912. At that time, protection from bacterial invasion was not adequate. During World War I, antiseptic procedures were found which made possible complete protection of the body from bacteria during operation. But no apparatus existed capable of playing the role of heart and lungs in keeping an organ alive and free from infection. This lack was supplied by the Lindbergh pump of 1935, with which life and function were preserved as long as the organs were perfused; the perfusion was carried on up to forty days.

It was found by microscopical and other tests that the structure and functions varied according to the chemical composition of the perfusing fluids. Thus it was made possible to dissect the body, as it were, into living parts and to learn that these parts adapt in vitro their morphological and functional activities to the condition of their medium. An indefinite number of tests of nutrient substances on isolated organs could be carried out and their effects determined. In this manner, Carrel believed the way was opened for the solution of many physiological and pathological problems.

In 1938, Carrel and Lindbergh published their book on the Culture of Organs. With this book, Carrel's career as an investigator may be said to have come to an end. In the book, he pointed out that machines are always in process of becoming, this process being almost unlimited; and he predicted that the cultivation of the whole organ had not reached its final form.

He saw the phenomena of growth, regeneration, wound healing, and hormone secretion rendered more comprehensible by studies of the effects of varied fluids diffusing from the capillaries into the tissues. And he cited, con amore, Claude Bernard, who said: "We will require a scientific explanation of the phenomena only when we are capable of determining, within the internal organic medium, the general conditions of nutrition by all histological elements, together with the nutrient agents specific to each of these elements."

Up to this point, Carrel's scientific work has been presented so as to show its logical development, beginning with his student days in the Lyon Hospital. But there is one episode which lies outside this order. Carrel was in France in 1914 when war broke out. He became associated at once with the military hospitals in Lyon, and soon with the Beaujon Hospital in Paris, where he carried out experiments on laboratory animals, with chemical disinfectants.

At the beginning of 1915, the Rond Royale Hotel at Compiegne was turned into a small military hospital for the severely wounded, and Carrel made its director. The hospital contained provision for research. Before it was opened to patients, H. D. Dakin joined Carrel, and prepared essentially neutral solutions of sodium hypochlorite buffered with borax and boric acid—the well-known Dakin solution—that was both germicidal and not too irritating to the tissues. The infected wounds were kept bathed in this solution by means of special surgical devices—called the Carrel technique—and under its influence infection could be controlled.

The treatment, which is known under the name of Carrel-Dakin, received wide endorsement at the time, was introduced later into civil surgical practice, and now, after thirty years, is being used in the present war.

EDITORS' NOTE

In his well-deserved Nobel Prize winning work, Alexis Carrel was half a century ahead of his time. By the end of the 1st decade of the 20th century he had perfected the techniques of modern vascular surgery and used them for successful transplantation of kidneys, hearts, small bowel and other organs. With the aviator Charles Lindbergh he developed a pump for perfusing organs that was the forerunner of cardiopulmonary bypass and organ preservation decades later. Carrel's pioneering tissue culture work was also important. But it was controversial.

Flexner cold not have known how wrong he was when in his memoir he endorsed Carrel's claim to have achieved the immortality for his cultured bits of chicken embryo hearts. Twenty five years later was it shown by Leonard Hayflick that the remarkably extended survival of Carrel's pulsating cardiac cells was either a laboratory error or a hoax. When in 1961 Hayflick found he could not repeat Carrel's results he performed experiments proving that normal cells cannot divide more than 20-40 times before they die. Thus Carrel's cardiac cells would have succumbed long before the 34 years he claimed. Carrel's technician later confessed that when the pulsating cells began to look puny to save them and please her boss, she added to the culture some fresh embryonic cardiac cells. Whether Carrel was aware of this (as some charged) we will never know.

What Flexner obviously did know but charitably left out of the memoir was an account of Carrel's last few years. As he had done during the 1st World War, during WWII Carrel again returned to his native France. This time with the blessings of the Vichy Government and the German occupiers, he headed a Foundation that studied and taught nutrition and demographics.

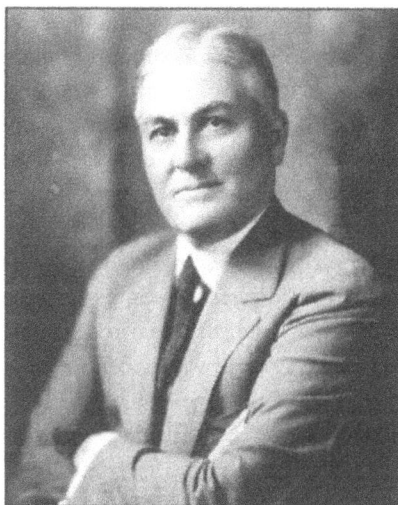

GEORGE WASHINGTON CRILE

1864–1943 (APS 1912)

Memoir by Evarts A. Graham

George Washington Crile, eminent surgeon, died in Cleveland, Ohio, on January 7, 1943, aged 79 years. He was born in Chili, Ohio, November 11, 1864, received an A.B. degree from Ohio Northern University in 1885 and the degree of M.D. from the University of Wooster Medical Department (now Western Reserve University School of Medicine) in 1887. He was Professor of Principles and Practice of Surgery, University of Wooster, 1893-1900; Professor of Clinical Surgery, Western Reserve University School of Medicine, 1900-11; Professor of Surgery, Western Reserve University School of Medicine, 1911-24. He received five honorary degrees, and he was given an honorary fellowship in eight foreign medical and surgical organizations. He was awarded numerous prizes and medals from American and foreign institutions, including the Lannelongue Medal of the Société Internationale de Chirurgie de Paris and the United States Distinguished Service Medal. He was elected a member of the American Philosophical Society in 1912.

Dr. Crile was one of the first to study the problem of surgical shock by experimental methods. Although some of his early conclusions were later shown by others to be untenable, his contributions did much to emphasize the importance of certain factors in the prevention of shock. At the time of his early investigations American surgery, under the influence of German thought and practice, was largely of a "rough and ready" sort, characterized by anesthesia which was atrocious from the modern viewpoint, a rough almost brutal handling of the tissues and but little regard for hemostasis.

Dr. Crile was chiefly responsible for the introduction of nitrous oxide into surgical practice, although its anesthetic properties had been discovered many years earlier. This was one of the most important contributions to the subject of practical surgical anesthesia that had been made in forty years. He early recognized the value of local anesthesia and upon its use he based some of his much discussed principles of "anoci-association." He was a constant proponent of sharp dissection and gentle handling of tissue at the operating table. His incessant emphasis on these points simultaneously with that of Halsted counteracted the German influence of rough operating. He early recognized the importance of hemostasis in the prevention of shock and was one of the first to foresee the practical importance of blood transfusion even before the knowledge of different blood groups had made it a feasible procedure.

Likewise, he was a pioneer in emphasizing the importance of the emotional factor in surgery. His plan of "stealing" the gland in toxic thyroid cases, by which the patient was lightly anesthetized two or three times before the day of operation and thus kept in ignorance of when it was to take place, was influential in avoiding the emotional stress of worry. Before the rediscovery of the effectiveness of iodine in controlling the toxic condition of such patients his plan undoubtedly contributed much in the accomplishment of his remarkably low operative mortality in this disease.

The gradual accumulation of knowledge of how to prevent surgical shock has been very largely an American contribution. In importance the solution of this problem ranks with asepsis and anesthesia. Crile's persistent emphasis on the problem and his own pioneer contributions to its solution places him as one of the most important creators of modern surgery. The earlier surgeons had been trained largely in anatomy and gross pathology. They had but little concern with function. Crile stood on the threshold of a new era, that of what might be called physiological surgery. It was perhaps more than a coincidence that at the age of twenty-six, three years after receiving his medical degree, he was appointed Professor of Physiology at the University of Wooster, a position which he held for three years. This early interest in physiology was maintained throughout his career.

Among his very numerous published papers and books there is almost nothing of the sort which distinguished the preceding leaders of surgery, practically no studies in the fields of human anatomy or pathology. The study of function, normal or pathological, was a consuming passion throughout his life. He was interested in the activities of a single cell, of an organ, of a human being and even of masses of human beings collected together into what is known as society.

His restless inquisitive mind, coupled with a remarkable energy, sometimes led him astray into fields which he was not adequately prepared to enter. But criticism never evoked any bitterness from him. Even his closest associates never saw any display of anger or heard him utter any derogatory remarks about anybody. He had a sharp appreciation of humor, but seldom related a humorous incident. Even his casual conversation revealed that his mind was constantly creative, that he was always thinking of newer and better ways in which to treat sick patients and sick society.

It was perhaps natural that so dynamic a personality as Crile should develop a never failing interest in the question of the mechanism of the transmission and expenditure of energy in the living animal. This interest led to an extensive comparative anatomical study of the sympathetic nervous system, the endocrine glands, the brain, the heart and blood volume of nearly 4000 animals representing almost all the known species of the Arctic, the temperate and the equatorial zones. As a part of this inquiry, he and Mrs. Crile made extensive trips to various regions of the earth which permitted Dr. Crile to obtain and to dissect fresh material on the spot. Much of this material is now on display in the Museum of the American College of Surgeons at Chicago.

The conclusions drawn from this study, which was published in 1941 in his book, Intelligence, Power and Personality in Man and Animals, were that the qualities named in the title of the book seem to be dependent on the absolute and relative sizes of the various organs mentioned. Thus the carnivorous animals, dependent upon their agility in catching their food, have much larger adrenal and thyroid glands and much more highly developed sympathetic nervous systems than the herbivorous animals.

Dr. Crile was regarded by all his colleagues as a master surgeon. His operating was brilliant and rapid, and he made numerous technical contributions to this art. One of his major interests was the improvement of the type of surgery to which the average person was exposed. He was one of the original group of twelve which founded the American College of Surgeons in 1912 for that purpose. He served as its president in 1916 and 1917, and he was the chairman of the Board of Regents continuously from 1913 to October 1939, when he requested that he be not considered as a candidate for re-election. Much of what the College has accomplished has been due to his unfailing and tireless interest in its welfare and the enormous expenditure of time and energy which he devoted to it.

In both the Spanish-American War and in World War I he volunteered his services. In 1915 he proposed the unit organization of American base hospitals which was adopted and continued in this war. The Lakeside Hospital Unit which he organized was the first to go overseas with our Army in 1917. He served not only as professional director of that unit, but subsequently as senior consultant in surgical research in France with the grade at first of lieutenant colonel and in November 1918, of colonel. In 1921 he was made brigadier general in the Medical Officers' Reserve Corps.

In 1921 he became one of the co-founders of the internationally known Cleveland Clinic Foundation and Hospital, to which he devoted most of his energy after resigning from his professorship of surgery. In spite of a disastrous fire only a few years after its establishment, this institution has become one of the outstanding private clinics of the world.

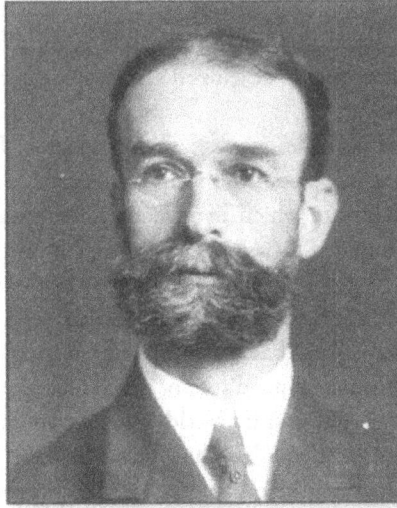

THEOBALD SMITH

1859–1934 (APS 1915)

Memoir by Edwin G. Conklin

In the death of Dr. Theobald Smith on December 10, 1934 the American Philosophical Society has lost one of its most distinguished members. Dr. Smith was born at Albany, New York, on July 31, 1859. He was graduated from Cornell University in 1881 where his associations with Professors Gage and Wilder gave him a life-long interest in general biological problems. He received the degree of M.D. from the Albany Medical School in 1883, and from 1884 to 1895 he was Assistant, and then Chief of the Division of Animal Pathology, Bureau of Animal Industry, Washington, D. C.

From 1886 to 1895 he was Lecturer and then Professor of Bacteriology in Columbia, now George Washington University, and from 1895 to 1914 was Professor of Comparative Pathology in Harvard University. In 1911–12 he was Exchange Professor from Harvard University to the University of Berlin. He was also Director of the Antitoxine and Vaccine Laboratory and Pathologist of the State Board of Health of Massachusetts from 1895 to 1914.

He was a member of the Board of Trustees of the Carnegie Institution of Washington and a Scientific Director of the Rockefeller Institute for Medical Research from its beginning in 1901, acting as Vice-President of the Board from 1924 to 1933 and succeeding the late Dr. William H. Welch as President in October 1933. In 1915 he organized the Department of Animal Pathology of the Rockefeller Institute at Princeton, New Jersey and served as its Director until his retirement in 1929.

Dr. Smith's researches on parasitism and disease were very extensive and of the most far-reaching importance; only a few of these can be mentioned here. With Dr. Salmon he demonstrated for the first time that killed cultures of bacteria may produce immunity; this is the principle now used in protective vaccination against typhoid, paratyphoid and cholera.

While in the Bureau of Animal Industry in Washington he demonstrated between 1888 and 1893 that ticks were the means of transmission of Texas cattle fever. This was the first proof ever given that insects may transmit disease germs and it opened the way to the discovery by others of the method of transmission of malaria, yellow fever, African sleeping sickness, etc. In 1896-'98 he proved that the bovine type of tubercle bacillus differed from the human type and this has played an important part in the present campaign against tuberculosis.

He first observed in 1904 cases of serum sickness and death in guinea pigs that had received a second injection of horse serum, and this hypersensitivity, which is akin to certain forms of asthma, hay fever, etc. in man, was at first known as the "Theobald Smith phenomenon." He demonstrated in guinea pigs the immunizing action of balanced or neutral mixtures of diphtheria toxine-antitoxine, and this method is now in general use as a preventive of human diphtheria. In addition to these and other discoveries bearing directly upon the causes and control of human diseases, Dr. Smith made many other studies on diseases peculiar to domestic animals, which for lack of time cannot be enumerated here.

Fortunately he had published only a few months before his death his Vanuxem Lectures for 1933 on "Parasitism and Disease," in which volume he summarized much of this work, and in which he emphasized especially the biological interrelationships of parasite and host. Indeed it may be said that it was his broad biological outlook and especially his confidence in the principle of organic adaptation between parasite and host that guided him in all his studies.

His really epoch-making discoveries brought him worldwide recognition and honors. He was a member of more than a score of the leading scientific societies of America and Europe, including the National Academy of Sciences of the United States, the Royal Society of London, the Royal Academy of Denmark, the Academy of Sciences of Paris, etc. He had been awarded by universities and scientific societies in this country and abroad eleven medals and twelve honorary degrees.

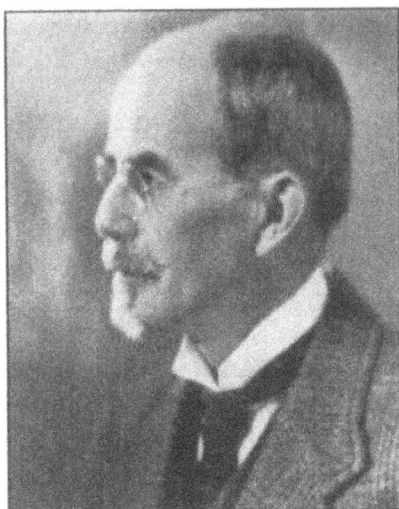

JOHN JACOB ABEL

1857–1938 (APS 1915)

Memoir by William H. Howell

Dr. Abel died in Baltimore on May 26, 1938 in his eighty-second year. He was at the time a patient in the Johns Hopkins Hospital for a slight ailment, but his death came unexpectedly from sudden heart failure. After his retirement in 1932 from the active duties of his position as Professor of Pharmacology in the Johns Hopkins Medical School he continued his investigative work as Director of the Laboratory of Endocrine Research, a position which was created for him largely through the generosity of the Carnegie Corporation. In spite of a somewhat frail physique and his advanced age he was constant in attendance at his laboratory during the academic year, although post mortem examination revealed that he suffered from serious cardio-vascular trouble that might well have incapacitated a less ardent worker.

Abel was born in Ohio, near Cleveland, on May 19, 1857, of German parents. His collegiate training was obtained at the University of Michigan from which he received the degree of Ph.D. in 1883. He was then twenty-six years of age, older, therefore, than the usual college graduate. The discrepancy is accounted for by the fact that during his college period there was an interim of three years during which he served as principal of a high school at La Porte, Indiana.

At graduation he was looking forward to a career in medicine and it is interesting that instead of remaining at Ann Arbor, where there was a good medical school and where it would have been relatively easy for him to make his degree, he decided to go to Germany, then the mecca for students of medicine who aspired to the best scientific training. It seems probably that he was influenced in arriving at this decision by the advice of Vaughan and Sewall who were then members of the medical faculty at Ann Arbor, and who subsequently became so well known as leaders in the modernization of American medical education.

However this may be Abel showed unusual wisdom and foresight in preparing himself for a career in medical science. From the beginning he sought a fundamental training on the chemical side, although the trend of opinion at that time was not in this direction. Ambitious young men looking forward to such a career were encouraged rather to acquire the techniques of the morphological and experimental laboratories. The great future of chemistry in its application to medical problems was not clearly envisaged, and indeed in this country at that time there was no medical school which could offer adequate courses in the subject.

Abel seems to have had from the beginning an understanding of the importance of the chemical approach and a determination to acquire the best training the world could afford. He spent seven years in Germany at various universities. While he studied under the leading masters of anatomy and physiology and did not neglect the clinical sides the greater portion of his time was given to the chemical aspects of physiology and pharmacology. He received his degree of M.D. from the University of Strassburg in 1888 and thereafter spent some time in practical clinical work in Vienna, under the impression that the outlook for a career in medical science in America was not promising, and that it might be necessary on his return to earn a living from the practice of medicine.

Actually this alternative was not forced upon him. He was fortunate enough, while working in Schmiedeberg's laboratory, to receive a call to a professorship in the medical school of the University of Michigan. Vaughan who was Dean had made up his mind to develop a modern department of pharmacology in the school such as did not then exist elsewhere in the country. He wrote to Schmiedeberg for suggestions for a suitable head, having in mind the importation of a German pharmacologist. Schmiedeberg advised against this plan and recommended Abel for the chair.

His advice was followed although Abel at that time had only his good training to offer as a guaranty of future performance. He was appointed Professor of Materia Medica and Therapeutics, and no better choice could have been made. While he remained at Ann Arbor only two years he inaugurated a department which in the hands of his eminent successors, Cushing and Edmunds, has become a leading center for pharmacological research.

When the medical school of the Johns Hopkins University was founded in 1893 Abel was called to the chair of pharmacology and was given charge also of the instruction in physiological chemistry, although his title this time was Professor of Pharmacology. It was probably the first chair under that designation established in this country.

It was during the forty years that he occupied this position that he did his great work in pharmacology and physiological chemistry and came to be recognized as the Father of American Pharmacology. He was the chief founder and first president of "The American Society for Pharmacology and Experimental Therapeutics." Together with Herter he was responsible for the establishment of The Journal of Biological Chemistry and in 1909 he started The Journal of Pharmacology and Experimental Therapeutics which he edited for twenty-three years.

Through these agencies and his own publications and the work of his advanced students he exerted a profound influence upon the development of pharmacology in this country. His own investigations were largely in the field of biological chemistry. His long training in chemical technique brought its reward when he undertook a study of the nature of the internal secretions.

His series of papers upon the chemistry of epinephrine aroused the interest of both chemists and physiologists and may be looked upon as the beginning of the brilliant contributions which have since been made to the subject of endocrine chemistry. His work on epinephrine, his crystallization of insulin and his method of studying the composition of the circulating blood by vividiffusion constitute his best known contributions. Each subject was the occasion for numerous papers.

The importance of his work is indicated by the many honors bestowed upon him by scientific societies and institutions. He received honorary degrees from the universities of Cambridge, Aberdeen, Lviv, Michigan, Pittsburgh, Harvard and Yale, and was awarded the Willard Gibbs, Conne and Kober medals and the medal of the Society of Apothecaries, London.

He was made a member of the National Academy of Sciences in 1912 and of the American Philosophical Society in 1915. On the day of his death he received news of his election as a Foreign Member of the Royal Society, London.

Abel had a genial lovable personality which inspired affection on the part of his students and friends. His outstanding characteristic, the one most frequently commented upon by those who knew him well, was his whole hearted devotion to scientific research. It was this ideal that sent him to Germany to get his training, and his contacts there with the masters in research, during the golden period of German medicine, served to intensify his enthusiasm. It was the moving principle in his life's work and no outside interest was permitted to divert him from his laboratory investigations.

While he managed very effectively to avoid commitments that tended to involve him in other activities he was always ready to give his time and energy freely to any movement that looked toward the promotion of scientific research. His zeal in this direction showed no abatement in his old age. It was recognized and appreciated by his fellow workers. Without conscious effort on his part he became one of the acknowledged leaders of medical research in this country.

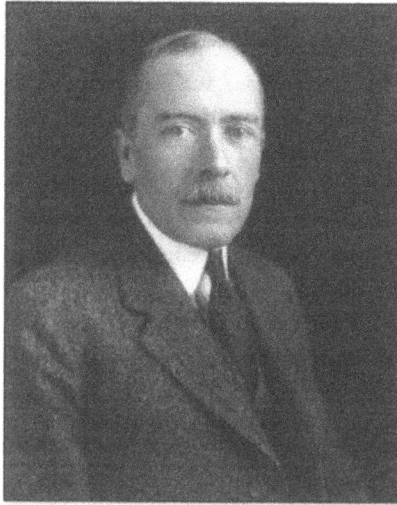

LIVINGSTON FARRAND

1867–1939 (APS 1923)

Memoir by Charles F. W. McClure

Livingston Farrand was born on June 4, 1867, in Newark, New Jersey. He received his early education in the Newark Academy, of which his father was headmaster, and spent a year in business before entering Princeton University, from which he graduated in 1888. He then attended the College of Physicians and Surgeons in New York City, receiving the degree of M.D. in 1891. The increasing interest which the study of physiological psychology was at that time receiving, especially in England and Germany, led Dr. Farrand to choose for specialization this subject, rather than the practice of medicine, and in preparation he spent two years in graduate study abroad in the Universities of Cambridge (1891–1892) and Berlin (1892–1893).

On his return to the United States, he joined the faculty of Columbia University. In the autumn of 1893 he became Instructor there in Physiological Psychology, in 1899 Instructor in Psychology, and in 1901 Adjunct Professor of Psychology. Meantime his interests were again taking a new direction; in 1903 he was appointed to the chair of anthropology, a position he held until 1914.

Soon after its formation in 1904, Dr. Farrand was made Executive Secretary of the National Association for the Study and Prevention of Tuberculosis. This was the first work he did in connection with welfare and philanthropic organizations, in the service of which his medical training and his extensive experience in dealing with problems of physiological psychology, psychology, and anthropology, were to prove so ideal a foundation. Under his nine-year administration of this office, branches of the tuberculosis association were formed in every state of the union and in our island possessions; enrollment in the National Association rose from 500 to 2256 members; and there was a corresponding increase in special tuberculosis hospitals, dispensaries, sanatoria, and open air schools.

The difficult question of providing financial support for all these was solved when he induced the Red Cross to turn over to tuberculosis work the entire income from the Christmas Seals; this provided a generous support and the seal itself carried with it, even to the humblest home, a sympathetic message of health and of the need of preventing the disease.

In 1914 Dr. Farrand resigned from Columbia to become President of the University of Colorado. During the five years that he served there, he worked energetically to revivify this institution and to establish its medical school on a sound basis. Soon his influence was felt far beyond the University, as is evidenced by the fact that he played a leading role in bringing to satisfactory settlement bitter labor disputes throughout the State of Colorado.

In 1917 the University of Colorado granted Dr. Farrand leave of absence to assist in war work. On account of his previous success in organization and his unique personal qualifications in dealing with difficult situations, he had been selected by the Rockefeller Foundation as the most suitable man to head the Commission it was sending abroad to assist the French in their attempt to control tuberculosis. In undertaking this mission, he knew he would be severely handicapped by an unfamiliar language and by the suspicions which France felt of all foreign offers; he was well aware also, that America had little to teach the land of Pasteur regarding the nature of tuberculosis. He is quoted as saying to President Poincaré, "We are not here to give you instructions, but to fight with you against a common enemy."

Through his tact, wisdom and statesmanship, and especially through his sensitiveness in understanding the attitude of those with whom he dealt, in less than two years he had established the French Anti-Tuberculosis Association and had won for the Commission the complete confidence of the French people. In recognition of his accomplishment, the French Government made him Officer in the Legion of Honor; twenty years later, he was made Commander. Among the distinguished achievements of Livingston Farrand, his contribution to the cause of tuberculosis control is perhaps the most striking.

From the beginning of the war, Dr. Farrand had been in close touch with the American Red Cross, which drew him to its service even during his work in France. Many months before the armistice, members of the War Council of the Red Cross had determined to spare no effort to preserve for time of peace the efficiency and high morale achieved in their work in time of war, and had been looking for a wise and vital leader who could hold together the forces of the Red Cross until these could be redirected to new and useful purposes.

Dr. Farrand was the first and only choice of the Council for this work and on their recommendation President Wilson appointed him Chairman of the Central Committee, to take charge on March 1, 1919. Mr. Eliot Wadsworth, Acting Chairman of the Red Cross, recently made the following statement: "The Red Cross today stands on the foundation so wisely designed and constructed by Dr. Farrand in the three critical years following the war. His wise knowledge of the problems of public health and social welfare enabled him to plan and develop a programme which did not conflict with existing agencies in these fields. His leadership maintained the high spirit of service, which, during the war, had made the Red Cross a great constructive force both nationally and internationally. He brought to the organization three priceless qualities—a keen sense of humor, an unusual ability to plan and organize, and dauntless enthusiasm which overrode all obstacles."

Dr. Farrand was called to the presidency of Cornell University in 1921. Under his administration of sixteen years, the university moved forward to substance, prestige, and influence. It was an organization of great complexity, comprising four state institutions, five endowed colleges, and a graduate school; but his fair-mindedness and magnanimity, his easy persuasive speech, and his engaging and disarming humor, enabled him to administer these with consummate tact, equity, and integrity.

He accomplished the task of uniting two strong but separated forces in New York City—the Cornell Medical School and the New York Hospital—into one great project devoted to medical education, service, and research; and one of the last of the many distinctions bestowed on Dr. Farrand was his appointment to membership on the Board of Governors of the New York Hospital, the first physician to be so recognized in one hundred and twenty-three years.

Dr. Albert R. Mann, who served with Dr. Farrand, first as Dean of the New York State College of Agriculture, and later as Provost of Cornell University, states: "Dr. Farrand's remarkable clarity of thought and expression, his sagacity and broad understanding, his manifest objectivity and his warm personality and unusual charm endowed his leadership of faculty and trustees with the confidence and devoted support of his associates. Courage, kindliness, and resourcefulness never failed him. These fortunate attributes, enriched by a contagious spirit and spacious sympathies, made his influence felt throughout the University. To an extraordinary degree, giving himself without reserve, he entered into the lives and activities of undergraduates, faculty, trustees, alumni, and the Ithaca community in which Cornell University is so happily placed. Cornell and Ithaca came to love this man deeply."

Some of the other positions held by Dr. Farrand show the wide scope of his interests and influence. He was a member of the Technical Board and of the Board of Trustees of the Milbank Memorial Fund; member of the Public Health Council of the State of New York; trustee of the American Museum of Natural History; Chairman of the Board of Trustees of the Carnegie Foundation for the Advancement of Teaching; Chairman of the World's Fair Committee on the Hall of Man; Director of the American Museum of Health. He was the recipient of eighteen honorary degrees from colleges and universities; he became a member of the American Philosophical Society in 1924.

Shortly after Dr. Farrand's death, which occurred on November 8, 1939, a memorial meeting was held in the New York Academy of Medicine, in recognition of his great service to humanity; on this occasion addresses were delivered by eleven speakers, representing twenty-two organizations and institutions with which Dr. Farrand had been closely associated. The memorial booklet containing these speeches pictures Livingston Farrand as the great public benefactor, the great educator, and the great gentleman that he was; they show that his personality was as perfect in its quality as his life was rich in accomplishment, and place him among the most eminent Americans of his time.

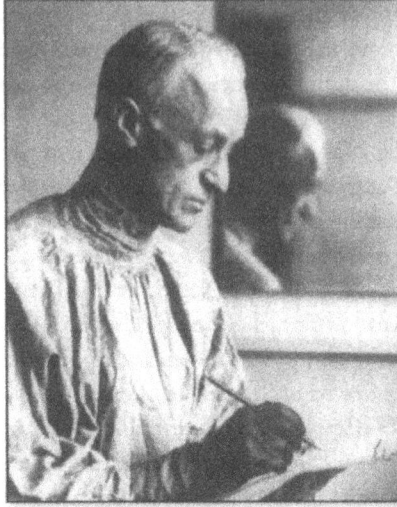

HARVEY CUSHING

1869–1939 (APS 1930)

Memoir by John Homans

Harvey Cushing came of old New England stock, a family mainly professional and of so enterprising a sort that in the early days of New England it left the East to aid in developing the Western Reserve of New Connecticut. When a man of this background turns out to be a genius, his nature is likely to be complex and stimulating. Such Cushing's was: intelligent, artistic, intense, untiring and ambitious. His traditions directed him into clinical medicine, a field to which he probably was best adapted, for he was always more an artist than a scientist.

His undergraduate training was at Yale University, his post-graduate education at Harvard University and the Massachusetts General Hospital. His early surgical years, those of his first, vigorous productive period, were passed at Johns Hopkins University. His truly scientific training came late, from Kocher, Kroneker and Sherrington. Thus, his clinical side was developed first and always predominated.

It was Cushing's fortune to fall in with Osler, a man whom he admired, loved and intuitively copied. From Osler, Cushing took his interest in books and writing, perhaps some part of his desire to inspire and help his younger professional colleagues. It is easy to see how the example of Osler's admirably shrewd and generous helpfulness influenced Cushing's more artistic and egotistical character. However, even Osler could hardly have improved Cushing's native quality as an observer or have shown him how to make a more picturesque record of his patients and their diseases. In effect, Osler directed Cushing's tastes in a direction likely to make them most productive, gave him a life-long avocation, and served as an example of teacher and clinician which Cushing always had in mind and often followed.

Viewed in this light, Cushing's career, a stirring, successful and well-rewarded one, was entirely logical. At Johns Hopkins University, Halsted was chief, brooking no rival. Much Cushing learned from him and carried this knowledge into that new field which his own vigor and imagination caused him to cultivate—the surgery of the nervous system. Here he attacked the brain tumor which hitherto had defied all attempts at cure or, for that matter, investigation.

His teaching and research were carried on at the Johns Hopkins Hunterian Laboratory, where he made his first fundamental observations upon the physiology and pathology of the pituitary gland. Indeed, during his entire subsequent career, he continued to make, on this subject, brilliant contributions which opened with his identification of asexual adiposity as a symptom-complex resulting from a lack of hypophyseal activity.

In Cushing's early forties, at the height of his mental and physical vigor, he created an atmosphere so brilliant and productive as to make him the obvious choice of Harvard University, for its Mosely Professorship in surgery, and of the newly opened Peter Bent Brigham Hospital, for its first Chief Surgeon. Actually, Cushing's appointment as Mosely Professor was only made two years after he had been invited to come to Boston, on the death of Dr. Maurice H. Richardson.

In Boston, he continued his development of neurological surgery and, here, there began to flock to him, from all over the world, young men who saw their opportunity to be introduced, under the most stimulating auspices, into a great new surgical field. What he was able to do for these men, and for others less bent upon specialization, is sufficiently told by their subsequent careers, almost universally successful. From Cushing, they learned, painfully, perhaps, at moments, the art of observation and of systematic recording, which left nothing to the imagination, but, above all, they were taught the most meticulous care of the patient—the gentle, safe performance and exquisite completion of formidable, dangerous, operative procedures, the painless and conscientious changing of complicated dressings.

Undoubtedly, Cushing's life as a professor of surgery and chief executive of the surgical department in a general hospital was not entirely happy. He was a first-rate judge of men but lacked in some degree the power to delegate authority. He stimulated rather than instructed. He neither readily entered into the ideas of others nor communicated to them his own. Had he been so endowed he could hardly have been the genius he was. Nor, as a scientist, was he entirely beyond criticism. That he made, from the clinic and laboratory, a more important contribution to medicine than any other man of his day is proved by the recognition he received from learned and scientific bodies all over the world, honorary degrees, honorary membership in famous scientific bodies without number.

Yet he was no Pasteur. He had brilliant ideas, brilliant conceptions of disease, which his inclination never tempted him to disprove, for he saw the confirmatory more clearly than the unfavorable evidence. In other words, he was an ardent human being and lacked the cold, critical faculty of the true scientist.

The sides of Cushing's teaching which his pupils and associates found most inspiring were the artistry and perfection of his operative technique, the minuteness of the study and care of his patients. The particular difficulties which he had had to face in searching for and removing brain tumors had led him to invent special procedures for dealing with soft and often excessively vascular tissues. The cotton pledgets, with black silk attached, the clips of silver wire for closing a blood vessel at the full reach of a narrow-bladed artery clamp, indeed, the elaborate rites, as they really were, of cerebral surgery, all were artistic to a degree.

The same artistry was evident in his case histories, which were filled not only with systematic preoperative data, photographs, sketches and charts, but, following his surgical therapy and as the years went on, with information derived from the patient, his family and his local physician, a complete story, in every last detail, of the subsequent life of the individual.

This nicety and unending care in the treatment of his patients and the study of their diseases is Cushing's contribution both to the art and science of surgery, a contribution so fundamental that no follower of his will ever be willing to depart from the principles that such a master has laid down.

Writing, with Cushing, was as important a side of his art as his clinical observations, operations and experimental work. It began with operative notes and sketches, which he would make, however tired he was, after his long hours of operating. His publications were intended to be authoritative, to be based upon a full knowledge of what others had done. They must refer to the important contributions of the past, the earlier fundamental contributions, especially if they were picturesque and of vital, human interest. They must be readable and, if possible, entertaining.

In writing, Cushing seldom dictated, and once having arranged his ideas on paper, mulled over and corrected his product until he was utterly satisfied. Although the result was polished, it was still vigorous and not at all self-conscious. Anyone who has ever seen one of Cushing's manuscripts will never forget it—the small handwriting, a little cramped, with its long letters gracefully curved—insertions, transpositions everywhere. Nor can one forget his sketches, vigorous, accurate, recording a dramatic moment of an operation or a patient's characteristic attitude.

Cushing's publications were mainly scientific, beginning with "The Pituitary Body and its Disorders," and ending with his superb, complete study, the "Meningiomas, Their Classification, Regional Behaviour, Life History and Surgical End-Results." Yet he felt impelled, and inspired, to write many essays which were published under the title of "Consecratio Medici," and his innumerable addresses and lectures would constitute for some literary men a life's work. For all this, he had time—it took several years—to write a biography of Sir William Osler, a complete, year-by-year story of a full life with all its personal contacts and interrelations with the world of medicine. He saw to it that the name of no one, whose associations with Osler contributed in any way to develop his character or illuminate his life, should be omitted. He made Osler live again in the recollection of everyone who at any time had met him. He was, indeed, a generous biographer.

Like many other intense persons, Cushing could relax in a delightful way. One evening, a young British surgeon, who was visiting him, suggested that they go to the circus. They did so and enjoyed themselves very well, but at the end of the show, Cushing was not quite satisfied. He suggested that they should look up some of the performers and see what they were like.

So off the two went, arm in arm. The circus was packing up, preparing to entrain itself for another city, and so the investigators ended their search in a freight yard at the car of the tattooed lady. Cushing had no particular knowledge of the circus, its performers in general or of tattooed ladies in particular, but was so charming and so sympathetic that a very interesting and sensitive woman gave them tea and told them the touching story of her life. It was like Cushing, that when he did embark upon a venture of this sort, his intellectual curiosity should continue active, with results impossible to foresee.

It was another of his attractive qualities that he should remember in detail and relate with gusto those experiences and incidents which appealed to his imagination and his whimsical sense of humor. No one was ever the worse for these stories, for he was never coarse or malicious. And since, in good company, he could listen as well as talk, he was in demand with groups of able and intellectual men who enjoyed meeting together, whether at table or elsewhere. In any gathering he was at once magnetic and provocative. He was elected to the American Philosophical Society in 1920.

Cushing's successful, productive years at Harvard University and the Peter Bent Brigham Hospital, years which made him the foremost figure of the medical world, were followed by his return to Yale University, his Alma Mater, which honored itself and him by freely offering him the opportunity to reflect, to follow up those patients whose course, as the years went on, must confirm or modify his conceptions of disease and treatment, to collect and publish his observations upon brain tumors, his clinical life's work, to write vigorous addresses, full of fascinating historical notices, and to continue the development and strengthening of his remarkable medical library.

It was altogether characteristic of him that in his last years, he sought out those great men, still living, who had made, during the last fifty years, the most striking and fundamental advances in all the sciences and secured from them reprints of their most famous work.

Shortly before his death, he had seen plans completed for a great medical library at Yale University, a library to which he had long looked forward to entrusting his most cherished possession, a superb collection of medical books. With the acquisition and study of these books are associated, as his intimates realize, many ingenious inquiries and researches unknown to the world. Of these adventures it was fascinating to hear him tell, and indeed, the atmosphere of his library best brought out those delightful qualities which made Harvey Cushing, to all who enjoyed his friendship, a beloved figure.

EDITORS' NOTE

This memoir benefits greatly from the personal touch provided by Harvey Cushing's colleague, John Homans. But even this excellent account ascribes less than the deserved importance to this giant of American medicine. He was truly one of the first of this country's physicians to be the world's leader in his field. Almost single handedly he invented modern neurosurgery. He trained the next generation of leaders in the field. Through his work on the pituitary gland he was a founder of endocrinology. In addition he was a noted bibliophile, a medical historian, a war hero, a skilled medical illustrator, and a writer who was awarded the Pulitzer Prize for the biography of his close friend, William Osler. He became so famous that the Queen Mary once held up it's sailing from New York to wait for Dr. Cushing who was delayed by cross town traffic. Those who desire to know more should read Michael Bliss' excellent 2006 biography, "Harvey Cushing; A Life in Surgery".

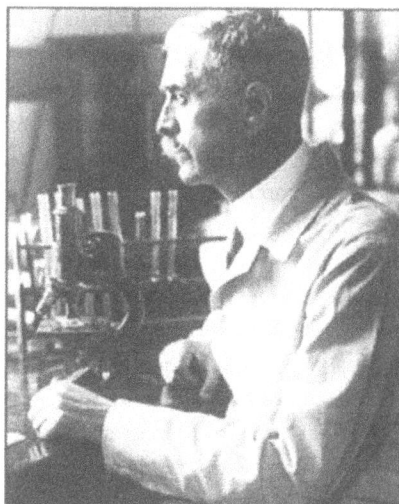

KARL LANDSTEINER

1868–1943 (APS 1935)

Memoir by Simon Flexner

Dr. Landsteiner was born in Vienna on June 14, 1868, and died in New York on June 26, 1943. Educated in Vienna, he took his medical degree in 1891, but instead of preparing himself for the practice of medicine he followed his stronger bent and fitted himself for the pursuit of a laboratory career as an investigator by devoting several years to the study of chemistry under Emil Fischer in Wurzburg, Bamberger in Munich, and Hantsch in Zurich.

The period was propitious for research in medicine; immunology was at the threshold of that development which was soon to become so spectacular and beneficent. Ehrlich and Bordet were launched on their remarkable careers, and Behring had already announced the discovery of diphtheria and tetanus antitoxins and had put them to practical test.

Returning to Vienna in 1897, Landsteiner first attached himself to the Hygienic Institute under von Gruber, one of the discoverers of the phenomenon of agglutination. There he spent only one year and transferred to the Pathological Institute under Weichselbaum, the discoverer of the meningococcus, with which Institute he remained connected during the rest of his years in Vienna, becoming professor extraordinarius of pathological anatomy in 1911.

In 1908, Landsteiner was appointed prosector (pathologist) to the Wilhelminen Hospital in Vienna. Thus until the fall and dismemberment of Austria after World War I, Landsteiner was engaged actively in teaching and research, and in the practical work of a hospital pathologist. In order to better his position and to improve his opportunities for scientific work, Landsteiner joined the staff of The Rockefeller Institute in 1922.

Among the earliest of Landsteiner's immunological studies were those which led to the discovery of the blood groups, a discovery which was thirty years later to bring him the award of the Nobel Prize. The investigation which yielded the knowledge of blood groups was not undertaken in haphazard fashion. Serological methods had already revealed that the proteins in various animals and plants are different and specific for each species. The multiformity is increased by the fact that also the various organs contain peculiar proteins.

The existence of biochemical species specificity prompted the question whether also the individuals within a species show similar, if only slighter, differences. No observations on this point existed. Landsteiner chose the simplest among the possible plans of investigation, as well as the material which gave promise of useful application. Accordingly, he allowed blood serum and blood corpuscles of different individuals to react one on the other. In some cases, no changes were observed; in others the reaction of agglutination or clumping of the corpuscles occurred.

The underlying facts of the blood groups had been discovered which further study separated into the four main groups which are the foundation of present-day blood transfusion. Landsteiner sensed the practical value of his discovery, although blood transfusion had long been abandoned.

The idea of treating disease by means of the transfusion of blood from a healthy to a sick person is an ancient one. The first experiments—showing this possibility—were carried out in Oxford. They began in 1658 with Sir Christopher Wren's infusion of medicated solutions into the veins of animals. Lower's classical experiment of passing blood direct from the artery of one dog into the veins of another was performed in 1665, and repeated in London before The Royal Society. Pepys records transfusion in his diary of 1666. In 1667, Denys of Paris transfused the blood of a lamb into a man, and later that year Lower and King carried out a human transfusion before The Royal Society.

But the occurrence of fatalities led to the prohibition of the practice in France, and these dangers, together with a long controversy involving theological as well as medical arguments, plunged the practice into neglect where it virtually remained until Landsteiner's discovery more than two hundred years later. But his discovery, which made transfusion a safe, life-saving operation, was not adopted immediately.

In 1907–08, Ottenberg carried out the first transfusion with matched blood, that is, the blood of the donor and the blood of the recipient having been proven compatible by the agglutination test. Even then transfusion was employed only occasionally. It was during World War I that it was resorted to frequently; and after the War, the practice became general throughout the world. It was after the wide recognition of the great medical value of blood transfusion that the Nobel Prize was awarded Landsteiner in 1930. Blood grouping has found other applications, as in forensic medicine for the determination of paternity and the identification of blood stains, and in studies in heredity and anthropology.

Although Landsteiner's name is primarily associated with the knowledge of blood groups, this discovery constitutes only a small share of the important and new work he accomplished. For example, to mention only two instances, his name is connected also with the mechanism responsible for the singular disease, paroxysmal haemoglobinuria, in which the organism breaks down no inconsiderable part of its own blood when a foot or arm is chilled, and with the transmission of poliomyelitis (infantile paralysis) to old world monkeys, the starting point of the many important investigations since made of that puzzling disease.

But immunology continued to be his main interest, and by 1914 he had formulated and entered on the task which was to occupy him for the rest of his life, and for which his peculiar talents and thorough training, both in chemistry and pathology, especially fitted him. The dominant idea of the long series of researches in this field carried out by Landsteiner and his pupils relates to the dependence of immunological phenomena on chemical structure.

Of the two main factors which enter into the immunity reactions, antigen and antibody, Landsteiner chose the former for study, for the reasons that antigens are available in quantity and in relative purity and lend themselves to the complex chemical manipulations which mold their chemical and biological characters. In 1921, he described the haptens, substances which, while capable of uniting with antibodies, are nevertheless incapable of giving rise to immunity.

Landsteiner's fruitful researches on the serological reactions, while primarily of theoretical nature, have also had important practical implications. It has been said of him that he found serology a mass of phenomena and he left it a branch of chemistry, and that his discovery of complex chemospecific antigens and the recognition of chemospecific anaphylaxis made possible the development of a general concept which is able to explain anaphylaxis, allergy, hypersensitiveness, and idiosyncrasy from the same or a similar point of view.

Dr. Landsteiner received the Paul Ehrlich Medal and the Gold Medal of the Dutch Red Cross Society. He was an honorary member of many societies and academies. He was elected a member of the American Philosophical Society in 1935.

www.ingramcontent.com/pod-product-compliance
Lightning Source LLC
Chambersburg PA
CBHW082147150426
42812CB00076B/2323